The Unholy Hymnal

Terminological Inexactitudes and Delusions
Rendered by
PRESIDENT RICHARD M. NIXON
VICE PRESIDENT SPIRO T. AGNEW
PRESIDENT LYNDON B. JOHNSON
VICE PRESIDENT HUBERT H. HUMPHREY
SECRETARY OF DEFENSE ROBERT S. MCNAMARA
SECRETARY OF DEFENSE MELVIN R. LAIRD
SECRETARY OF STATE DEAN RUSK
SECRETARY OF STATE WILLIAM P. ROGERS
GENERAL MAXWELL TAYLOR
GENERAL WILLIAM C. WESTMORELAND
ATTORNEY GENERAL JOHN N. MITCHELL
FBI DIRECTOR J. EDGAR HOOVER
and
Other Choirboys of the Credibility Gap

Compiled by
ALBERT E. KAHN
with the assistance of STEVEN *and* BRIAN KAHN

WOLFE PUBLISHING LIMITED
10 EARLHAM STREET
LONDON WC2

ISBN 72340448 8

Printed by C. Nicholls & Company Ltd
The Philips Park Press, Manchester

*To those members of the press
and of other communications media
who have revealed crucial truths
to the American public
during the era of the Credibility Gap*

The political lie has become a way of bureaucratic life. It has been called by the more genteel name of "news management." I say here now, let's call it what it is—lying.

> Walter Cronkite,
> speech before Inland Press Association
> February 23, 1966

In order to avoid the embarrassment of calling a spade a spade, newspapermen have agreed to talk about the "Credibility Gap." This is a polite euphemism for deception . . .

> Walter Lippmann
> March 28, 1967

The government has become attuned to falsehood as a routine way of conducting its affairs. Official lies on matters large and small, foreign and domestic, are the daily fare of the Washington press corps.

William McGaffin and Erwin Knoll
Anything But the Truth, 1968

. . . Senators have been misled so many times in the last five years by what the Administration said it was doing in Vietnam that many of them simply do not believe what they are told.

James Reston
New York Times
February 5, 1971

Every aspect of the war is layered over by mistruth, misinformation, misstatement and silence. None of this lying and hiding has a jot to do with military security. . . . It's done to conceal graft, stupidity, bad judgement from our own people; it's done in the hopes that you can execute policies in secret that you wouldn't dare to attempt if they were known.

Nicholas Von Hoffman
Washington Post Service
February 27, 1971

Contents

Foreword

ON GOVERNMENT BY MISREPRESENTATION

It is likely that most Americans, wishing to respect their nation's leaders, are reluctant to think of them as liars. This perhaps accounts for the politely euphemistic tone of the phrase "Credibility Gap," which was coined in the mid-1960's and has since become indispensable to our vocabulary.

In previous periods of American history, as Walter Lippmann has noted, there seems to have been no need for such a phrase. That is not of course to say that the nation's former leaders always told the truth. The Cold War years preceding the Johnson Administration had, in fact, yielded a rich variety of governmental deceits. The very concept of defending a Free World that included a fascist Spain, military dictatorships in Latin America, and a feudal oligarchy on Formosa placed a certain strain on credulity. Nor was public confidence fortified by such events as the U-2 incident, when what was, according to the Government's version, a civilian plane on a weather research flight over Turkey proved to be a CIA plane on a spy mission over Russia; or by the Bay of Pigs episode, when the Government first denied any part in the invasion and then admitted having masterminded the whole operation. As a matter of fact, the Assistant Secretary of Defense for Public Affairs, Arthur Sylvester, publicly declared in 1962 that in times of crisis the Government had "the right to lie" to the people; and in view of the prevailing world tensions, American officials perhaps already considered this "right" a perennial privilege.

But with the advent of the Johnson Administration, the full-scale involvement of the United States in the Vietnam war, and the growing dominance of the military-industrial complex, the falsities and fictions of officialdom underwent both a quantitative and qualitative change. Never before had they proliferated in such abundance or with such abandon. Grotesque fabrications, patent untruths and specious fantasies assumed an almost routine character; no subject was too serious, or too insignificant, for distortion or camouflage. Commenting upon an instance of the State Department's falsifying the facts about peace negotiations with Hanoi, a White Paper prepared by the Senate Republican Policy Committee declared in 1967, "This episode, when added to the host of other incidents, utterances, misleading statements, half-truths, outright untruths, emphasizes the hallmark of the Johnson Administration in the conduct of the Vietnam war—a complete lack of candor." Nor has the hallmark changed under the Republican Administration of President Nixon. By early 1971, according to a Gallup poll, some 70 percent of the American people believed that the Government was deliberately misinforming them about the situation in Vietnam. Misrepresentation seems to have become a matter of government policy.

Under our laws, lying under oath can be a criminal offense, punishable by fines and imprisonment; and though high government officials do not swear to tell the truth when they take their oaths of office, one might question the logic of permitting them to deceive with impunity the citizenry they have sworn to represent. They may of course contend that the deception of the public is in the public interest; but when their falsehoods imperil the lives and welfare of millions, their offense seems graver than that of the private citizen who perjures himself.

The purpose of this book is to provide a compendium of the falsities and delusions that have emanated from government officials—and their colleagues in the military-industrial complex—during the era of the Credibility Gap. There have been hundreds of untruths for each one cited; but it is hoped that this selection, though fractional, may serve as a handbook providing a useful record of the recent past and a warning for the immediate future.

The passages in color that intersperse the text intend to contrast the fictions with the facts of this period. Most of these passages record events that time has proven to be part of reality; some, which may be said to be statements of opinion, reflect truths the author believes self-evident in the light of current events. Not all may completely provide instant refutation of the falsities that precede them; rather, it is the cumulative effect of both which is most conclusive.

A hymnal format seems appropriate for the presentation of the medley of misleading voices, because of their generally pious tone. No irreverence is intended toward those noted hymns from which the chapter titles have been borrowed. Conceivably, some of the nation's leaders might consider this hymnal irreverent toward *them*. But when the President, the Vice President and the Attorney General use such terms as "bums," "garbage," and "stupid bastards" to describe a sizable portion of the population, they themselves can hardly object to being characterized simply as liars.

I should perhaps emphasize that not all of the falsities assembled here are necessarily conscious deceits. Purveyors of untruths can delude themselves into believing their own fantasies. It is, I suppose, quite possible that not infrequently the President and his top associates actually believe they are telling the truth. And there is, of course, no simple formula for deciphering the mechanics or motivations of these governmental minds. The reader must decide for himself which of the untruths cited in this book are outright lies, deliberate deceits, subterfuges, half-truths, hyperboles, incredible misjudgments, pure fatuities, or mere delusions.

ALBERT E. KAHN
May 1971

NOTE: *This book was completed and being set in type when on June 13, 1971,* The New York Times *began publishing the secret Pentagon Papers with their disclosures regarding the origins and conduct of the war in Indochina. The* Times *exposé will doubtless assist the reader in determining which of the governmental statements recorded in my chapters on Indochina are outright lies or mere delusions. I have made no changes in the book, other than including occasional footnote references to the Pentagon study, listing it among useful source references, and commenting on it in the Epilogue.*

A.E.K.
July 1971

Book One

Hymns of Indochina

1

Lord, Let Us Now Depart in Peace

In which keeping the peace is the reason given for waging war, and each extension of the war is said to be the means of ending it

With dignity and conviction

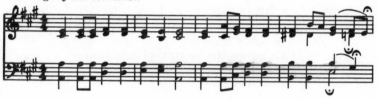

Our constant aim, our steadfast purpose, our undeviating policy; is to do all that strengthens the hope of peace.

President Lyndon B. Johnson
Los Angeles, California
February 24, 1964

U.S. TO ENLARGE VIETNAM FORCE
BY 5,000 ADVISERS—TOTAL TO BE 21,000
New York Times
June 21, 1964

Peace ought to be possible in Southeast Asia without any extension of the fighting.

> Secretary of State Dean Rusk
> Washington, D.C.
> June 30, 1964

U.S. PLANES ATTACK NORTH VIETNAM BASES:
PRESIDENT ORDERS "LIMITED" RETALIATION
AFTER COMMUNISTS' PT BOATS RENEW RAIDS
> *New York Times*
> August 5, 1964

Our one desire—our one determination—is that the people of Southeast Asia be left in peace to work out their own destinies in their own way.

> President Johnson
> On signing the Tonkin Gulf Resolution*
> Washington, D.C.
> August 10, 1964

I have had advice to load our planes with bombs and to drop them on certain areas that I think would enlarge the war and result in committing a good many Americans to fighting a war that

---

* *The Tonkin Gulf Resolution, which virtually authorized President Johnson to wage war—without declaration of war—in Vietnam, was passed by Congress at the President's request following the "deliberate and unprovoked attack" on two U.S. destroyers by North Vietnamese torpedo boats on August 4, 1964. Neither of the U.S. vessels showed any signs of damage after the alleged attack.*

"Subsequent investigations," writes Colonel James A. Donovan in his book Militarism, U.S.A., *"revealed that there is considerable reason to doubt that an attack . . . did, in fact, take place."*

Tom Wicker of the New York Times *reported that President Johnson "had been carrying around for weeks" a draft of the Tonkin Resolution prior to the alleged attack. The Resolution was finally repealed in January, 1971.*

The secret Pentagon study which the Times *began publishing in June 1971 reveals that from late 1963 the U. S. had conducted "an elaborate program of covert military operations against the state of North Vietnam" and that part of this program was provocations designed "to provide good grounds to escalate [into overt war] if we wanted to."*

I think ought to be fought by the boys of Asia to protect their own land. And for that reason I haven't chosen to enlarge the war.

> President Johnson
> Stonewall, Texas
> August 29, 1964

As the United States has frequently stated, we seek no wider war.

> White House statement announcing
> air raids over North Vietnam
> February 7, 1965

U.S. JETS ATTACK NORTH VIETNAM
IN REPRISAL FOR VIETCONG RAIDS
New York Times
February 8, 1965

Today peace in Southeast Asia can be obtained if the violators will cease their aggression.

Our policy is clear. . . .

We seek no wider war. . . . Our goal in Southeast Asia is to-day what it was in 1954—what it was in 1962. Our goal is peace and freedom for the people of Vietnam.

> Vice President Hubert H. Humphrey
> United Nations General Assembly
> New York, N.Y.
> February 17, 1965

I regret the necessities of war have compelled us to bomb North Vietnam. . . . The people of South Vietnam and the Americans who share their struggle suffer because they are the attacked, not because they are attackers.

> President Johnson
> Washington, D.C.
> April 17, 1965

For months during the [election] campaign, the Administration line was that the war in South Vietnam was substantially self-sustaining and had to be won there. Almost overnight, when the bombing of North Vietnam began, information was produced to prove that "aggression from the north" . . . is the key to everything.

> Editorial
> *New York Times*
> April 30, 1965

. . . he [President Johnson] had made the momentous decision to bomb North Vietnam nearly four months earlier . . . it can now be revealed, in October, 1964, at the height of the Presidential election campaign. . . . But he also had good reasons for delaying the execution of his decision . . . the problem of working with a stable South Vietnamese government . . . the problem of preparing for the bombing raids. . . .

These were the only reasons for delay the President mentioned when he told me in May, 1965, that he had made the decision to bomb four months before Pleiku.* But it is fair to assume there were other considerations: One certainly was the fact that the United States was engaged in an election campaign. . . . The American public . . . was not prepared psychologically for a deliberate calculated step-up in the war effort.

> Charles Roberts
> *LBJ's Inner Circle*, 1965

* A raid by Vietcong guerrillas on the American base at Pleiku on February 7, 1965, served as President Johnson's justification for launching sustained bombing raids against North Vietnam. The Pentagon Papers published in June, 1971 confirm Charles Roberts' account that the bombings were planned months in advance. The Pentagon study also indicates that a major reason for delaying them was the "tactical consideration" that President Johnson was campaigning for election as a self-proclaimed candidate of reason and restraint as opposed to the avowedly hawkish Barry Goldwater.

QUESTION: What do you regard as the most important achievement of your four years in office?

SECRETARY OF STATE RUSK: The steady reduction of the causes of war.

Interview in *Newsweek*
May 17, 1965

There has been no change in the mission of the United States ground combat units in Vietnam in recent days or weeks. . . . The primary mission of these troops is to secure and safeguard important military installations.

White House statement
June 9, 1965

U.S. ADDING 21,000 TO VIETNAM FORCE
The reinforcements will bring American military strength . . . to a total of 70,000 or 75,000 men.

New York Times
June 17, 1965

JOHNSON ORDERS 50,000 MORE MEN
TO VIETNAM AND DOUBLES DRAFT
New York Times
June 29, 1965

So peace—peace, that simple little five-letter word—is the most important word in the English language to us at this time and it occupies more of our attention than any other word or any other subject.

President Johnson
Washington, D.C.
August 25, 1965

21

MORE U.S. TROOPS AND PLANES
DUE TO GO TO VIETNAM
New York Times
November 12, 1965

Peace is more within our reach than at any time in this century. . . .

President Johnson
Omaha, Nebraska
June 30, 1966

U.S. EXTENDING BOMBING,
RAIDS HANOI AND HAIPHONG OUTSKIRTS
New York Times
June 30, 1966

U.S. VIETNAM FORCE TO BE AT 475,000 IN '67
New York Times
November 21, 1966

NAVY IS SEEKING TO WIDEN ATTACKS
ON NORTH VIETNAM
New York Times
December 12, 1966

QUESTION: Does it remain American policy not to bomb Hanoi?
STATE DEPARTMENT PRESS OFFICER, ROBERT J. MCCLOSKEY: It is not American policy to bomb other than . . . military targets or militarily associated targets.

QUESTION: Well, could these militarily associated targets be located within the city limits of Hanoi?

MCCLOSKEY: I don't know what the city limits are.

State Department Press Conference
Washington, D.C.
December 14, 1966

Tonight . . . I am taking the first steps to de-escalate the conflict. We are reducing—substantially reducing—the present level of hostilities.

> President Johnson
> announcing partial bombing halt over North Vietnam
> Washington, D.C.
> March 31, 1968

The "de-escalated" U.S. bombing campaign over North Vietnam, now restricted to supply lines below the 20th parallel, actually is more intensive than it was before the March 31 restriction went into effect. Bombing sorties over the southern panhandle of North Vietnam during April are expected to run well over 7,000; there were 5,000 in March over the whole of North Vietnam. . . .

> *Newsweek*
> May 6, 1968

I pledge you tonight that the first priority foreign policy objective of our next Administration will be to bring an honorable end to the war in Vietnam. . . . My fellow Americans, the dark long night for America is about to end.

> Former Vice President Richard M. Nixon
> Presidential Nomination acceptance speech
> Republican National Convention
> Miami, Florida
> August 8, 1968

My own view is that President Johnson set in motion the processes of peace [in Vietnam] and Mr. Nixon is going to reap the harvest.

> Former Vice President Hubert H. Humphrey
> Washington, D.C.
> February 20, 1969

QUESTION: Mr. President, there's been growing concern, sir, about deepening U.S. involvement in Laos. If you could confirm that, would you also say whether this runs counter to your new Asian policy?

PRESIDENT NIXON: There are no American combat forces in Laos. . . .

QUESTION: Mr. President, you say there are no combat forces in Laos. How do you regard the airmen who bomb the Ho Chi Minh trail from bases in Thailand and Vietnam? Would you regard those as combat forces?

PRESIDENT NIXON: . . . we do have aerial reconnaissance, we do have, perhaps, some other activities.

News Conference
Washington, D.C.
September 26, 1969

There are no American combat troops in Laos.
President Richard M. Nixon
Washington, D.C.
March 7, 1970

WASHINGTON (CDN)—Tens of thousands of Americans have engaged in combat activities in the secret war in Laos. . . .

The United States has spent more than a billion dollars on the war—almost all of it in secret.

These are some of the key facts to emerge with the publication of the Senate Foreign Relations Committee testimony taken at closed hearings on Laos. . . .

Essentially, testimony shows, the Nixon administration has concealed the dimensions of the aerial war by emphasizing the relatively small number of U.S. personnel actually based in Laos. This figure is no more than 2000. Yet this 2000 represents only a tiny fraction of those involved in combat activities in Laos, because most of those engaged in combat haven't been stationed in the country.

James McCartney
San Francisco Sunday Examiner & Chronicle
April 26, 1970

LAIRD ADMITS GI'S DO GO INTO LAOS
San Francisco Chronicle
May 19, 1970

Officials in the White House, the Pentagon and the State Department . . . strongly reaffirmed the United States policy of not widening the war in Vietnam. They said the rules of engagement had not been changed to allow American forces to penetrate Cambodia.

New York Times
March 28, 1970

It seems to us that our best policy is . . . to avoid any act which appears to violate the neutrality of Cambodia.

Secretary of State William P. Rogers
Report to Foreign Relations Committee
April 2, 1970

We finally have in sight the just peace we are seeking.

President Nixon
San Clemente, California
April 20, 1970

We recognize that if we escalate and we get involved in Cambodia with our ground troops our whole program is defeated.

Secretary of State Rogers
Testimony before House Appropriations
    Subcommittee
April 23, 1970

NIXON SENDS COMBAT UNITS INTO CAMBODIA
TO ATTACK COMMUNIST STAGING AREA
New York Times
May 1, 1970

This is not an invasion of Cambodia. . . . We take this action not for the purpose of expanding the war into Cambodia but for the purpose of ending the war in Vietnam, and winning the just peace we all desire.

President Nixon
Washington, D.C.
April 30, 1970

The assurances that the American-backed South Vietnamese drive into Cambodia is a limited, one-strike operation, an integral part of American operations in Vietnam and designed only to protect American and "free world" forces there, have a familiar and wholly unconvincing ring.

Editorial
New York Times
May 1, 1970

America's purpose in Vietnam and Indochina remains what it has been—a peace in which the people of the region can devote themselves to development of their own societies, a peace in which all the people of Southeast Asia can determine their own political futures without outside interference.

President Nixon
Washington, D.C.
June 30, 1970

U.S. SAYS PLANES
HIT HANOI REGION TO COVER MISSION
PENTAGON CONCEDES ATTACK AFTER DAYS OF DENIAL
New York Times
November 28, 1970

Disingenuous is a charitable word to describe Defense Secretary Laird's explanation of why he failed to tell the Senate Foreign Relations Committee that the November 21 bombing of North Vietnam included air strikes in the Hanoi area. "I only answer the questions that are asked," he said.

A sharper characterization was employed by Senator Fulbright, when asked in a television interview if Mr. Laird had been "candid."

"They misrepresent the facts. Obviously, he did, and they do it all the time," Mr. Fulbright said.*

> Editorial
> *New York Times*
> December 3, 1970

"The only American activity in Cambodia after July 1," President Nixon assured the nation last June, "will be air missions to interdict the movement of enemy troops and material where I find that is necessary to protect the lives and security of our men in South Vietnam."

. . . as long ago as last August reports from the field made it clear that the United States airmen were going well beyond "interdiction" to furnish close fire support to faltering Cambodian ground forces. Now, with . . . American aircraft openly committed in support of South Vietnamese and Cambodian troops battling to reopen a key highway from the sea to Pnompenh, the Pentagon has taken off the wraps and disclosed the Administration's intention to employ the full range of its air power in Cambodia.

> Editorial
> *New York Times*
> January 21, 1971

* As House Minority Leader during Johnson's Presidency, Representative Laird had frequently attacked the Administration for misrepresenting the facts in connection with the war in Vietnam. "The fault," he declared on April 30, 1966, "lies in great part with an administration that fails to inform the people fully and frankly about the objectives and progress of the war."

Last evening the Government of the Republic of Vietnam announced in Saigon that elements of its armed forces have crossed the enemy-occupied territory of Laos to attack North Vietnamese forces and military supplies which have been assembled in sanctuaries close to the border of South Vietnam.

This limited operation is not an enlargement of the war.

From the text of a State Department statement
February 8, 1971

WASHINGTON, Feb. 9—. . . Mr. Laird, who had appeared before the Senate and House Armed Services Committees, insisted to reporters on Capitol Hill that the Laos operation, rather than widening the war, as critics have asserted, has shortened it.

William Beecher
New York Times
February 10, 1971

NIXON REFUSES TO RULE OUT WIDER AIR ROLE
IN THE WAR OR A SAIGON PUSH TO THE NORTH
New York Times
February 18, 1971

I rate myself a deeply committed pacifist.

President Nixon
Interview with Cyrus Sulzberger
New York Times, March 9, 1971

2

𝔉𝔦𝔤𝔥𝔱 𝔱𝔥𝔢 𝔊𝔬𝔬𝔡 𝔉𝔦𝔤𝔥𝔱

*In which, amid claims of victory,
there is mounting evidence of defeat*

Triumphantly

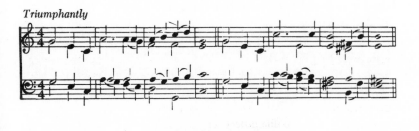

I can safely say that the end of the war is in sight.

> General Paul D. Harkins
> U.S. Commander, South Vietnam
> Tokyo, Japan
> October 31, 1963

In the entire week, I did not talk to a single official who was unable to agree that, if the proper effort is made, the war can be won.

> Secretary of Defense Robert S. McNamara
> reporting on visit to South Vietnam
> Washington, D.C.
> March 13, 1964

29

The military, economic, social and information programs together with the various technical programs have indeed built the springboard of victory.

> Former Ambassador to South Vietnam
> Henry Cabot Lodge
> Quoted in *Newsweek*
> January 18, 1965

Editors of this country do object to the contradictions, the double talk and half truths that the press is getting both in Washington and Saigon. . . .

The people of the United States deserve to be well informed in this crisis no matter how negative the news may be.

We fear it is not getting the full story nor the true story at this time.

> George Beebe
> President of Associated Press
> Managing Editors Association
> Miami, Florida
> April 20, 1965

The high hopes of the aggressor have been dimmed, and the tide of battle has turned.

> President Johnson
> New York, N.Y.
> February 23, 1966

The tide of battle has turned.

> Vice President Humphrey
> Washington, D.C.
> February 24, 1966

AMERICAN MILITARY DEATH TOLL IN VIETNAM PASSES 5,000 MARK

> *New York Times*
> October 16, 1966

There doesn't seem to be any clear direction to our military activities; we don't seem to be getting anywhere.

> Editorial, *Wall Street Journal*
> November 14, 1966

During the past year tremendous progress has been made. . . . We have pushed the enemy farther and farther back into the jungles. . . . We have succeeded in obtaining our objectives.

> General William C. Westmoreland
> Commander, U.S. Forces in South Vietnam
> Washington, D.C.
> July 13, 1967

A military machine tries to justify its role. Gen. Westmoreland, seeking indices of progress, will cite enemy casualties. Authorities have been stating for years that the guerillas are demoralized, have been denied recruits and are ineffective. Yet the enemy seems as obstinate and daring as ever. It breaks up big concentrations of American troops and scatters them by staging battles that burst like blisters across the anatomy of Vietnam.

> Dispatch from Saigon by AP correspondents
> Peter Arnett and Horst Fass
> Quoted in *I. F. Stone's Weekly*
> July 17, 1967

The other side is hurting and they are hurting very badly.

> Secretary of State Rusk
> Washington, D.C.
> July 19, 1967

I have never been more encouraged in my four years in Vietnam.

> General Westmoreland
> Washington, D.C.
> November 15, 1967

We are winning. It is pretty obvious that about all the enemy can do is resort to guerrilla tactics in large parts of the country and wait for an opportunity to take on our big units near his border sanctuaries.

> Admiral U.S. Grant Sharp
> Commander in the Pacific
> Honolulu, Hawaii
> November 21, 1967

VIETCONG ATTACK 7 CITIES
New York Times
January 30, 1968

FOE INVADES U.S. EMBASSY—
VIETCONG WIDEN ATTACK ON CITIES
New York Times
January 31, 1968

Our best experts think that they [the Vietcong] had two purposes in mind [in the Tet offensive].

First was a military success. That has been a complete failure. That is not to say that they have not disrupted services. It is just like when we have a riot in a town . . . or bridges go out, or lights—power failures and things. . . . A few bandits can do that in any city in the land. . . .

> President Johnson
> Washington, D.C.
> February 2, 1968

All week long . . . South Vietnam lay pinned in the grip of the bloodiest single convulsion the war has yet produced. After months of confident American predictions that the enemy was on the run, the Communists staged their boldest military stroke—

an astonishingly well-coordinated guerrilla offensive against the
supposedly secure cities of South Vietnam.

> *Newsweek*
> February 12, 1968

U.S. VIETNAM CASUALTIES
PASS THOSE OF KOREAN WAR
> *New York Times*
> March 15, 1968

Make no mistake about it—we are going to win.

> **President Johnson**
> **Minneapolis, Minnesota**
> **March 18, 1968**

In effect, the Americans are back where they were 18 months
ago. They are holding onto the towns and their own military
bases but, as far as the countryside goes, they are capable of little
more than mobile defense. . . .

In the light of what one sees in Vietnam, and of what everyone
there knows, some recent Pentagon statements . . . read as if
they had been drafted by Lewis Carroll.

> Dispatch by David Leitch
> in London *Sunday Times*
> Quoted in *San Francisco Chronicle*
> March 21, 1968

**Militarily we have never been in a better relative position in
South Vietnam.**

> **General Westmoreland**
> **Washington, D.C.**
> **April 7, 1968**

33

Vietcong and North Vietnamese opened a series of mortar and rocket attacks in Saigon and in cities and military bases throughout South Vietnam this morning.

> *New York Times*
> May 5, 1968

The enemy has been defeated at every turn.

> General Westmoreland
> Saigon, South Vietnam
> June 9, 1968

More Americans were killed in combat in the first six months of this year than in all of 1967, official figures showed today.

> *New York Times*
> July 4, 1968

Our forces have achieved an unbroken string of victories. . . .

> General Earle G. Wheeler
> Chairman, Joint Chiefs of Staff
> Washington, D.C.
> August 31, 1968

We have the enemy licked now. He is beaten. We have the initiative in all areas. The enemy cannot achieve a military victory; he cannot even mount another offensive. . . . In recent months General Abrams has taken the offensive from the enemy in a brilliant fashion.

> Admiral John S. McCain
> Commander in Chief in the Pacific
> Article in *Reader's Digest*
> February 1969

159 RAIDS STAGED BY FOE IN VIETNAM
FIGURE IS LARGEST SINCE TET DRIVE IN '68

> *New York Times*
> May 13, 1969

. . . I think history will record that this may have been one of America's finest hours, because we took a difficult task and we succeeded.

> President Nixon
> addressing troops
> Dian, South Vietnam
> July 30, 1969

FOE ATTACKS 100 CENTERS ACROSS SOUTH VIETNAM
New York Times
August 12, 1969

I judge that we are on the right track.

> General Wheeler
> Saigon, South Vietnam
> October 7, 1969

ENEMY IN VIETNAM OPENS WIDE DRIVE
ALLIES REPORT THE HEAVIEST CASUALTIES IN 8 MONTHS
New York Times
April 2, 1970

Tonight, American and South Vietnamese units will attack the headquarters [in Cambodia] for the entire Communist military operation in South Vietnam.

> President Nixon
> Washington, D.C.
> April 30, 1970

Based on General Abrams' report, I can now state that this has been the most successful operation of this long and difficult war. . . .

As of today I can report that all our military objectives have been achieved.

> President Nixon
> Report to the Nation
> on progress of Cambodia campaign
> Washington, D.C.
> June 3, 1970

In terms of military objectives, the main points made by the President in his speech of April 30 announcing the action were two: that the enemy was "concentrating his main forces in the sanctuaries where they are building up to launch massive attacks on our forces," and that in the eastern border areas of Cambodia there was "the headquarters for the entire Communist military operation in South Vietnam."

The headquarters has not been found; hardly anyone believes any more that it existed. Nor did our invading armies find the slightest evidence of Communist troop concentrations prepared for a "massive" attack on South Vietnam; virtually no enemy troops were in the border areas.

> Anthony Lewis
> *New York Times*
> June 6, 1970

U.S. RESCUE FORCE LANDED WITHIN 23 MILES OF HANOI BUT IT FOUND P.O.W.'S GONE

> *New York Times*
> November 24, 1970

We caught them completely by surprise.

> Secretary of Defense Melvin R. Laird,
> commenting on raid on prisoner-of-war camp
> November 24, 1970

SENATOR FULBRIGHT: I don't like to say it was all a bad idea simply because it failed, but it did fail. There was something wrong with the intelligence.

SECRETARY OF DEFENSE LAIRD: This was not a failure, Mr. Chairman. . . . This mission was carried on by a group of men that performed the mission with 100 percent excellence.

SENATOR FULBRIGHT: The men performed perfectly, but whoever directed it didn't, I mean. . . .

SECRETARY OF DEFENSE LAIRD: I would like to tell you, Mr. Chairman, that we have made tremendous progress as far as intelligence is concerned.

SENATOR FULBRIGHT: You mean since Friday?*

> Hearing before Senate Foreign
> Relations Committee
> November 24, 1970

The operation [in Laos] has been going very well.

> Secretary of Defense Laird
> Washington, D.C.
> February 17, 1971

> INVASION BOGGING DOWN—
> HEAVY RED OPPOSITION
> *San Francisco Examiner*
> February 22, 1971

I have been disturbed by reports, usually attributed to a junior officer in the field, that this operation has bogged down.

> Lieutenant General Vogt
> Pentagon briefing
> Washington, D.C.
> February 24, 1971

---

* *The raid on the empty prisoner-of-war camp took place on Friday, November 20.*

37

The operation is going according to plan.
> Secretary of Defense Laird
> Washington, D.C.
> February 24, 1971

HEAVY RED ATTACKS PERIL INVASION— HEAVY SOUTH VIET LOSSES
San Francisco Chronicle
February 27, 1971

SAIGON GI's REEL UNDER RED ATTACK
San Francisco Chronicle
March 19, 1971

Contrary to reports that you noticed in the last day or so in the papers, this was not a rout. This was an orderly retreat.
> **Vice President Spiro T. Agnew**
> **Newton, Massachusetts**
> **March 19, 1971**

2,000 TROOPS LEAVE LAOS PURSUED BY HANOI UNITS
New York Times
March 22, 1971

DESPERATE SAIGON SOLDIERS SCRAMBLE FOR HELICOPTERS
New York Times
March 22, 1971

WASHINGTON, March 22—Secretary of Defense Melvin R. Laird said today that the South Vietnamese drive in Laos was still "going forward according to plan."
> *New York Times*
> **March 23, 1971**

WASHINGTON—U.S. officials believe South Vietnamese forces in Laos have proved that they have "passed a milestone in their development" that will help assure continued withdrawal of U.S. forces from Indochina, President Nixon said Monday.

> Don Irwin
> *Los Angeles Times*
> March 23, 1971

U.S. PLANES COVER SOUTH VIET RETREAT

> *Los Angeles Times*
> March 23, 1971

We cannot judge it [the Laos campaign] before it is concluded, and we cannot judge it even after it is concluded.

> President Nixon
> Quoted in *Newsweek*
> March 29, 1971

3

𝕭𝖑𝖊𝖘𝖙 𝕭𝖊 𝖙𝖍𝖊 𝕿𝖎𝖊 𝕿𝖍𝖆𝖙 𝕭𝖎𝖓𝖉𝖘

*In which, while the avowed U.S. aim of Vietnamization
is that of aiding an ally to aid himself,
the assistance to him grows
as his self-sufficiency diminishes*

Rather slowly

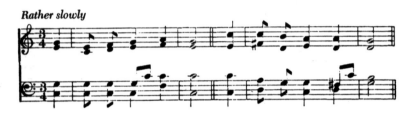

We have completed the job of training South Vietnam's armed forces.

> General Charles J. Timmes
> Commander U.S. Military Assistance Advisory Group
> in South Vietnam
> Tokyo, Japan
> October 31, 1963

We continue to be hopeful that we will be able to complete the training responsibilities of many of the United States personnel now in Vietnam and gradually withdraw them over the period between now and the end of 1965.

. . . We are only assisting them [the South Vietnamese] through training and logistical support.

> Secretary of Defense McNamara
> Testimony before House Armed Services Committee
> January 27, 1964

I don't know what the U.S. is doing. They tell you people we're just in a training situation. . . . But we're at war. We are doing the flying and the fighting. . . .

How our Government can lie to its people—it's something you wouldn't think a democratic government could do.

> From a letter of
> Air Force Captain Edwin Gerald Shank, Jr.,
> written to his wife shortly before
> he was killed on an air-strike mission
> *U.S. News & World Report*
> May 4, 1964

. . . we are not about to send American boys nine or ten thousand miles away from home to do what Asian boys ought to be doing for themselves.

> President Johnson
> Akron, Ohio
> October 21, 1964

The regular South Vietnamese forces have been considerably strengthened by the continuing flow of equipment. . . . The combat performance of regular troops continues to inspire confidence.

> Secretary of Defense McNamara
> Statement before House Armed Services Committee
> February 19, 1965

SAIGON' FORCE BATTERED
TOLL FOR 4-DAY ENGAGEMENT
PUT NEAR 900, A RECORD
New York Times
June 13, 1965

They're fighting well. They're fighting hard. They're fighting effectively.

> Secretary of Defense McNamara
> commenting on South Vietnamese
> troops, Washington, D.C.
> June 16, 1965

SENATOR STEPHEN M. YOUNG: The desertion rate of the South Vietnamese a year or so ago, I understand, was quite high. Is the desertion rate decreased? . . .

GENERAL HAROLD K. JOHNSON (Chief of Staff, U.S. Army): . . . There has been an improvement in the course of last year in the desertion rate.

> Testimony before Senate Armed Services
> and Appropriations Committee hearings
> January 24, 1966

About 96,000 men deserted from the South Vietnamese armed forces last year. . . . Desertions from the regular armed forces nearly doubled the last year.

> Neil Sherman
> *New York Times*
> February 24, 1966

In my first weeks as Secretary of Defense I have devoted most of my energies to a comprehensive review of our policies and programs with respect to Vietnam. Among the more important conclusions which emerged from that effort was that the South Vietnamese were ready to bear an increasing share of the military burden in the future and thereby enable us to level off and in due time begin to reduce our contribution.

> Secretary of Defense Clark M. Clifford
> Testimony before House Armed Services Committee
> April 30, 1968*

SAIGON REPORTS RISE IN DESERTION RATE**
New York Times
June 5, 1968

U.S. OFFICERS IN VIETNAM
DEPLORE PULLOUT TALK—
FEAR A PUBLIC COMMITMENT MAY BRING ON
COLLAPSE OF MORALE IN SAIGON REGIME
New York Times
June 7, 1969

What I was told and what I saw there persuaded me that "Vietnamization" is in fact a canopy being hoisted to shelter—perhaps to conceal—our staying in, not getting out. . . . I found no prominent American or South Vietnamese who thought the present

---

* *Shortly after testifying that "the South Vietnamese were ready to bear an increasing share of the military burden" and thus effect a reduction of the U.S. war effort, Secretary Clifford visited South Vietnam. What he found there he revealed a year later, after retiring from office. In the July 1969 issue of Foreign Affairs, Clifford wrote: ". . . I found little evidence that . . . the South Vietnamese were ready to relieve us of our burdens. . . . I returned home oppressed by the pervasive Americanization of the war; we were still giving the military instructions, still doing most of the fighting, still paying most of the bills. Worst of all, I concluded that the South Vietnamese leaders seemed content to have it that way." Significantly, on Clifford's return to the United States, he failed to make his findings publicly known.*
** *The desertion rate in the first three months of 1968 was up 40% from 1967. A total of 143,000 soldiers deserted from the South Vietnamese Army in 1968.*

government of South Vietnam would be able to maintain itself even in two or three years if our armed support were withdrawn.

Representative Allard Lowenstein,
on return from visit to South Vietnam
Washington, D.C.
September 24, 1969

WASHINGTON, Oct. 9—Secretary of Defense Melvin R. Laird said today that American commanders in South Vietnam were operating under formal new orders in placing the "highest priority" on shifting the burden of the fighting to the South Vietnamese.

Working under these new instructions since August, field commanders "have achieved a real momentum," Mr. Laird said.

William Beecher
New York Times
, October 10, 1969

. . . Secretary Laird's optimism has a familiar ring. For example, in December, 1965, Secretary of the Army Brucker said: "With a little more training, the Vietnamese Army will be the equal of any army."

Editorial, *New York Times*
October 13, 1969

President Nixon has a program to end the war. That program is Vietnamization.

Secretary of Defense Laird
Washington, D.C.
October 29, 1969

We are moving on schedule on Vietnamization.

President Nixon
Washington, D.C.
January 30, 1970

REPORT FOR SENATE UNIT ISN'T SURE
SOUTH VIETNAM CAN EVER ASSUME BURDEN
New York Times
February 2, 1970

The morale and self-confidence of the Army of South Vietnam is higher than ever before.

President Nixon
Washington, D.C.
June 30, 1970

SAIGON DESERTIONS UP NEARLY 50% IN SPRING*
New York Times
July 27, 1970

Vietnamization is working well.

Vice President Agnew
San Diego, California
September 11, 1970

The Central Intelligence Agency has told President Nixon that the Vietnamese Communists have infiltrated more than 30,000 agents into the South Vietnamese Government in an apparatus that has been virtually impossible to destroy.

Neil Sheehan
New York Times
October 19, 1970

* *The average monthly desertion rate from the South Vietnamese Army, reported this dispatch from Saigon, was about 8,000 in 1969; the number of deserters had risen to more than 11,000 in May 1970 and to nearly 12,000 in June.*

The Vietnamization program is moving forward with encouraging results.

> Admiral Thomas H. Moorer
> Chairman, Joint Chiefs of Staff
> Detroit, Michigan
> November 9, 1970

. . . tonight I can report that Vietnamization has succeeded.

> President Nixon
> Washington, D.C.
> April 7, 1971

4

Glorious Things
of Thee Are Spoken

In which a series of military dictatorships,
waging civil war under U.S. supervision,
are hailed as popular governments
seeking democratic reforms

With exultation

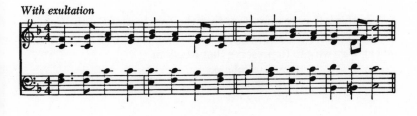

We believe that the present regime [in South Vietnam] has
moved promptly to consolidate public support . . .
>Secretary of State Rusk
>Washington, D.C.
>November 8, 1963

**VIETNAM JUNTA OUSTED BY MILITARY DISSIDENTS
WHO FEAR "NEUTRALISM"**
>*New York Times*
>January 30, 1964

47

General [Nguyen] Khanh . . . has in his first thirty days in office done much to build the support of the people.

> Secretary of Defense McNamara
> Washington, D.C.
> March 15, 1964

SAIGON, South Vietnam—Vietnamese observers say a coup against Premier Maj. Nguyen Khanh is only a matter of time. . . . General Khanh is concerned enough to sleep in a different house each night, to admit to foreign correspondents that his wife is worried and to house her and their four children 350 miles from Saigon.

> *New York Herald Tribune*
> April 19, 1964

We think it very important that the freedom of South Vietnam be preserved. . . . we are going to advise them and help them in every way we can to preserve that freedom.

> President Johnson
> Washington, D.C.
> April 21, 1964

The truth, which is being obscured from the American people, is that the Saigon government has the allegiance of probably no more than 30 percent of the people and controls (even in daylight) not more than a quarter of the territory.

> Walter Lippmann
> April 21, 1964

General Khanh is on the right track . . .

> Secretary of State Rusk
> Washington, D.C.
> April 21, 1964

KHANH QUITTING . . .

> *New York Times*
> April 21, 1964

We want . . . only that the people of South Vietnam be allowed to guide their own country in their own way.

> President Johnson
> Baltimore, Maryland
> April 7, 1965

OUR ALLY: A PREMIER WHOSE HERO IS HITLER

"People ask me who my heroes are. I have only one—Hitler." These are the words of Air Vice-Marshal Nguyen Cao Ky, latest Prime Minister of South Vietnam. . . .

We met in his huge office at Tan Son Nhut air base on the outskirts of Saigon, when Ky commanded the Vietnamese air force. . . .

Ky said: "I admire Hitler because he pulled his country together when it was in a terrible state in the early Thirties. But the situation here is so desperate now that one man would not be enough. We need four or five Hitlers in Vietnam."*

> Brian Moynahan
> *Sunday Mirror* (London)
> July 4, 1965

There is little evidence that the Vietcong has any significant popular following in South Vietnam.

> Secretary of State Rusk
> Washington, D.C.
> April 23, 1965

On March 3, 1966, at a public lecture at Cornell University, the Vietnamese Ambassador to the United States, Vu Van Thai, in clarification of Ky's earlier statement about Hitler, quoted the Premier as saying: "I want to infuse in our youth the same fanatacism, the same dedication, the same fighting spirit as Hitler infused in his people."

SAIGON—The Vietcong has achieved a high degree of immunity. They move freely through most of the country with little fear that the local populace will betray them.

Tom Ross
Chicago Sun-Times
May 23, 1965

. . . the mission of the Vietcong forces, the guerrilla forces, is to kill and terrorize the people, whereas the mission of the Government forces is to protect the populace.

Secretary of Defense McNamara
Washington, D.C.
June 16, 1965

BANMETHUOT, South Vietnam—Undisciplined South Vietnamese troops have been terrorizing the civilian population here in the Central Highlands. . . .

Troops have been looting the villages of mountain tribesmen, stealing from bars, stores and restaurants in towns, brawling in the streets, and robbing inhabitants at gunpoint.

Neil Sheehan
New York Times
September 18, 1965

The Administration is placing renewed hope on the possibility of a strengthened village pacification program in South Vietnam, tied in with Premier Ky's recent pledge to institute new, far-reaching social reforms.

New York Herald Tribune
February 5, 1966

U.S. AID KEEPS MAKING VIETNAMESE RICH RICHER
Washington Star
February 5, 1966

I think there is a tremendous new opening here for realizing the dream of the Great Society in the great area of Asia, not just here at home.

Vice President Humphrey
CBS "News Special"
Quoted in *New York Times*
April 20, 1966

South Vietnam is increasingly coming to grips with the need to modernize its society, bolster its civil economy, develop its representative institutions, and provide a better life for its people.

From a report released by the White House
September 13, 1966

Twelve years have elapsed since we began contributing economic assistance and manpower to South Vietnam. Yet that nation continues to face political instability . . . and to suffer . . . severe economic dislocations. Inflation continues to mount, . . . land reform is virtually nonexistent, agricultural and education advances are minimal . . .

From a supplement to a report of the
House Foreign Operations Subcommittee
October 12, 1966

Today's leaders in Vietnam, Chief of State Thieu and Prime Minister Ky, have given their solemn pledge that they will support the outcome of fair elections, whoever wins. . . .

In South Vietnam today, there are eleven candidates for President—some military, some civilian. They are free to attack the Government, and some have done so.

They are free to take their case to the people, and most have done so.

President Johnson
Washington, D.C.
August 16, 1967

President Johnson said today that South Vietnam had made more progress toward constitutional government in 13 months while fighting a war than the United States made in the first 13 years after the American Revolution.

New York Times
November 10, 1967

SAIGON, South Vietnam, Friday, July 26—Truong Dinh Dzu, the peace candidate who ran second in the presidential election last year, was sentenced today to five years of hard labor for having urged the formation of a coalition government as a step toward peace.*

New York Times
July 26, 1968

BIENHOA, South Vietnam, Aug. 27— . . . [President Nguyen Van] Thieu . . . emphasized strongly once again that his Government has ruled out negotiations with the National Liberation Front and the formation of a coalition government. . . .

"I would never accept any Communist to run in an election in Vietnam," he said. . . . "When we say one man, one vote, we mean the vote would be given to Vietnamese citizens who deserve it."

Bernard Weinraub
New York Times
August 28, 1968

QUESTION: Mr. Secretary, you have spoken repeatedly . . . about the importance of self-determination for South Vietnam and an open political process there. I wonder how you would reconcile this with the recent jailing of the Buddhist monks and the continued presence in prison of Truong Dinh Dzu, the presiden-

* In sentencing Truong Dinh Dzu, the judge of the military court in Saigon which had tried him stated: "As a citizen of the Republic of Vietnam, you have no right to dissent on the policy of the Government of the Republic of Vietnam."

tial candidate. Have you discussed this with the government of South Vietnam? What is your position on it?

SECRETARY OF STATE ROGERS: Yes, we've discussed it. I don't think the two questions are particularly related. One involves civil liberties and the other involves voting rights.

Press Conference
Washington, D.C.
April 7, 1969

The Thieu-Ky government is a military government propped up by American power, despised and corrupt. Freedom of speech is suppressed. No one knows how many Vietnamese political prisoners languish in Vietnam's prisons, but the figure is certainly in the thousands and includes university professors, religious leaders, lawyers, students, newspaper editors, politicians—anyone who has dared to advocate political initiatives to end the war.*

From a White Paper on Vietnam
issued by the American Friends Service Committee,
inserted in the *Congressional Record*,
May 7, 1969

SAIGON—A broad spectrum of South Vietnamese politicians believe that the present government of President Thieu is too weak, too narrow, too inept and too corrupt to compete successfully for power with the National Liberation Front. . . . Interviews with the most important political parties, fronts and religious blocs did not turn up a single individual who believed that the present

---

* *Among the numerous accounts of the tortures suffered by political prisoners under Thieu's regime, and the barbaric conditions of their confinement, was a widely publicized report by Representatives Augustus F. Hawkins of California and William R. Anderson of Tennessee, in July, 1970, of their visit to the Con Son Prison with its infamous "tiger cages."*

Thieu government could win a reasonably fair and open competition with the Communists.

> Peter J. Krumps
> *Baltimore Sun*
> June 2, 1969

When asked about Vietnam, Mr. Nixon celebrated President Thieu as a very capable man and excellent politician. . . . He called Mr. Thieu probably one of the four or five best political leaders in the world.[*]

> *New York Times*
> August 1, 1969

Deputy Defense Secretary David Packard concluded a 6-day assessment of the war effort today. . . . He praised South Vietnam's "remarkable progress" toward democracy.

> *New York Times*
> November 22, 1969

ZURICH (Reuters)—The International Press Institute today devoted the last section of its annual review of press freedom to South Vietnam. . . . The review said, "The bleakest prospect for press freedom is, paradoxically, in the country where a war is being waged in the name of freedom—South Vietnam. . . . The government does not hesitate to take ruthless action against the press and pressmen. . . . Numerous publications were suspended for varying periods throughout the year.

> *Baltimore Sun*
> January 2, 1970

[*] *President Nixon's evaluation of Thieu as a statesman was reminiscent of tributes to Premier Ngo Dinh Diem before his despotic regime was overthrown in 1963. Diem was acclaimed by Senator Hubert Humphrey as the United States' "best hope in South Vietnam" and by Vice President Johnson as "the Winston Churchill of Asia."*

5

𝕺𝖓𝖜𝖆𝖗𝖉, 𝕮𝖍𝖗𝖎𝖘𝖙𝖎𝖆𝖓 𝕾𝖔𝖑𝖉𝖎𝖊𝖗𝖘

*In which, while holy moralities are preached,
unholy monstrosities are practiced*

With martial rhythm

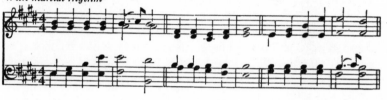

I've got on my watch the Golden Rule: "Do unto others as you would have them do unto you."
> President Johnson
> Quoted in *U.S. News & World Report*
> January 6, 1964

To see freedom sent around the world, this is our mission. . . . It was God's charge to us."
> Senator Barry Goldwater
> Quoted in *Newsweek*
> September 21, 1964

Of course, we act out of enlightened self-interest . . . But the pages of history can be searched in vain for another power whose pursuit of that self-interest was so infused with grandeur of spirit and morality of purpose.

> President Johnson
> New York, N.Y.
> October 14, 1964

In the past few weeks photographs have appeared in the British press showing the torture inflicted on Viet Cong prisoners by the Vietnam army. . . . The strange new feature about the photographs . . . is that they have been taken with the approval of the torturers and published over captions that contain no hint of condemnation. . . . These photographs are of torturers belonging to an army which could not exist without American aid and counsel. Does this mean that the American authorities sanction torture as a means of interrogation?

> Graham Greene
> *London Daily Telegraph*
> November 6, 1964

One of the most infamous methods of torture used by the government is partial electrocution—or "frying" as one U.S. adviser called it. . . . Sometimes the wires are attached to the male genital organs, or to the breasts of a Vietcong woman prisoner. . . . Other techniques . . . involve cutting off the fingers, ears, fingernails or sexual organs of another prisoner. Sometimes a string of ears decorates the wall of a government military installation.

> Beverly Deepe, from Saigon
> *New York Herald Tribune*
> April 25, 1965

Only the Vietcong has committed atrocities in Vietnam.
> **Vice President Humphrey**
> **Pittsburg, Pennsylvania**
> **May 13, 1965**

As battle rages we will continue as best we can to help the good people of South Vietnam enrich the condition of their life.

President Johnson
Washington, D.C.
July 28, 1965

Few Americans appreciate what their nation is doing to South Vietnam with airpower. . . . This is strategic bombing in a friendly, allied country. . . . significant numbers of innocent civilians are dying every day in South Vietnam.

Charles Mohr from Saigon
New York Times
September 5, 1965

Friend is often indistinguishable from foe. Napalm and fragmentation bombs sometimes fall on defenseless peasants; artillery shells are fired at random into the paddy fields. An appalling number of victims are women, children and old men; some are participants but most are noncombatants.

William Tuohy
New York Times Magazine
November 28, 1965

The U.S. Government has always abided by the humanitarian principles enunciated in the Geneva conventions and will continue to do so.

Secretary of State Rusk
in a letter to the
International Committee of the Red Cross, Geneva
August 10, 1965

. . . Secretary of State Dean Rusk informed the International Committee of the Red Cross in Geneva that the United States

. . . had plans to help South Vietnam create adequate facilities and procedures for handling of prisoners.

Neil Sheehan, from Saigon
New York Times
September 30, 1965

Many a news correspondent or U.S. Army military adviser has seen the hands whacked off prisoners with machetes. Prisoners are sometimes castrated or blinded. . . . The subjects of interrogation so often die under questioning that intelligence seems to be a secondary matter.

Malcom W. Browne
The New Face of War, 1965

As far as the United States Military Assistance Command in Vietnam is concerned, one mishap—one innocent civilian killed, one civilian wounded, or one dwelling needlessly destroyed—is too many. . . . We will not and cannot be callous about these people.

General Westmoreland
Washington, D.C.
August 26, 1966

And if there's any doubt . . . here at home about our purpose in Vietnam, I never find it reflected in those letters from Vietnam.

Our soldiers and our marines and our airmen and our sailors know why they are in Vietnam.

President Johnson
New York, N.Y.
February 23, 1966

Dear Mom and Dad:

Today we went on a mission and I am not proud of myself, my friends or my country. We burned every hut in sight.

. . . a buddy of mine called "La Dai" ("Come here") into a

hut and an old man came out of the bomb shelter. My buddy . . .
threw a hand grenade into the shelter. . . .

After the explosion we found the mother, two children (ages
about 6 and 12, boy and girl) and an almost newborn baby. . . .
The three of us dragged out the bodies onto the floor of the hut.

It was horrible!

The children's fragile bodies were torn apart, literally muti-
lated. We looked at each other and burned the hut. . . .

> From a letter from an American soldier,
> published in *Akron Beacon Journal*
> March 27, 1967

In the recent attacks on petroleum facilities, every effort has
been made to prevent harm to civilians and to avoid destruction
of nonmilitary facilities. The petroleum facilities attacked were located away from the population centers of both Hanoi and Haiphong. The pilots were carefully instructed to take every precau-
tion so that only military targets would be hit.

> Ambassador Arthur J. Goldberg
> New York, N.Y.
> June 30, 1966

It stood to reason that many North Vietnamese civilians lost
their lives yesterday, since bombs and exploding oil tanks are not
so exclusively accurate as to blow up in a vacuum or kill only
soldiers. As the British Government's statement of "regret" and
"disassociation" said, the bombs touched "on the populated areas
of Hanoi and Haiphong."

> Editorial
> *New York Times*
> June 30, 1966

I have followed our activity in Vietnam very closely. I think that the country knows, and I would like to repeat again, that it is the policy of this government to bomb only military targets.

President Johnson
Johnson City, Texas
December 31, 1966

What are the non-military targets that have been bombed? They are several residence areas in Hanoi, substantial areas of mixed housing, small shops and miscellaneous buildings in the suburbs of Gialam, Yenvien and Vandlien in the Hanoi metropolitan area, several schools in the Hanoi area, villages and hamlets along highways leading south from Hanoi, large areas of housing and shops in towns like Namdinh and Ninbinh and in the Phatdiem village complex, and a variety of other objectives, including cemeteries.

Harrison E. Salisbury
New York Times
January 13, 1967

You've got to forget about this civilian stuff. Whenever you drop bombs, you're going to hit civilians . . .

Barry Goldwater
New York, N.Y.
January 23, 1967

Now, as to bombing civilians, I would simply say that we're making an effort that is unprecedented in the history of warfare that we do not. . . .

President Johnson
Nashville, Tennessee
March 15, 1967

By mid-1966, more than 100,000 houses or huts had been destroyed from the air; by the end of 1966, the number will probably have reached 200,000. In other words, about one-fifth of all

South Vietnamese housing will have been razed. Seventy percent of the destruction is in the "liberated zones" of the NLF.*

> Kuno Knoebl
> *Victor Charlie*, 1967

We must be willing to continue our bombing until we have destroyed every work of man in North Vietnam if this is what it takes to win the war.

> General Curtis LeMay
> United States Air Force (Ret.)
> Long Beach, California
> April 1, 1967

Many communities in Vietnam are living a better life because of the encouragement and help our American troops have given to them. A true missionary zeal among our troops is commonplace and is one of the unique characteristics of this war.

I am constantly impressed by the concern for the lives of others shown by the men of my command.

> General Westmoreland
> New York, N.Y.
> April 24, 1967

One technique is to move into a Vietcong area, remove all the people to resettlement villages, and burn and destroy what remains.

But at least one-third of Vietnam's 15 million population would have to be resettled for this policy to succeed. . . .

---

* *In his book* Militarism, U.S.A., *Colonel James A. Donovan writes: ". . . at the end of October, 1968, when bombing of the North halted, the total bomb tonnage dropped in both North and South Vietnam was given as 2,948,057 tons. (Total tonnage dropped by U.S. aircraft in World War II, in both European and Asiatic theaters, was 2,057,244.) So we dropped almost 50 percent more bombs on Vietnam than in both Europe and the Pacific."*

Nevertheless, this "scorched earth" technique is the main one being used in the Vietnam war now.

Christian Science Monitor
April 4, 1967

Mr. McNamara said napalm was not indiscriminately used in Vietnam. Rather, he said, it is used with precautions that are as painstaking as we can make them without hamstringing our military operations.

New York Times
December 9, 1967

I have been an orthopedic surgeon for a good number of years. . . . But nothing could have prepared me for my encounters with Vietnamese women and children burned by napalm. It was sickening, even for a physician, to see and smell the blackened flesh. . . . And one never forgets the bewildered eyes of the silent, suffering napalm-burned child.

Dr. Richard E. Perry
"Where the Innocent Die"
Redbook, January 1967

It became necessary to destroy the town to save it.

U.S. Army Major,
referring to Ben Tre, South Vietnam
AP dispatch
February 7, 1968

We have dropped twelve tons of bombs for every square mile of North and South Vietnam. Whole provinces have been substantially destroyed. More than 2,000,000 Vietnamese are now homeless refugees.

Senator Robert F. Kennedy
Washington, D.C.
February 8, 1968

The American attitude toward the war is wholesome.
                    General Westmoreland
                    New Orleans, Louisiana
                    September 10, 1968

The peace we seek . . . is not victory over any other people, but the peace that comes with healing on its wings, with compassion for those who have suffered, with understanding for those who have opposed us . . .
                    President Nixon
                    Washington, D.C.
                    January 20, 1969

It has been more than a year since the rhetoric of peace began in Vietnam. During this time scores of thousands of men, women and children have died in the fighting. . . .

The human situation today in Vietnam is worse than it has ever been. An entire nation is being destroyed and the tempo of destruction has increased. One third of the rural people of this rural nation have become refugees. Hundreds of thousands of acres have been defoliated, countless villages have been razed. . . . The American Friends Service Committee, which has been involved in the relief of war suffering for more than half a century, has rarely encountered such misery as in Vietnam today.
                    From a White Paper on Vietnam
                    issued by the American Friends Service Committee,
                    inserted in the *Congressional Record*
                    May 7, 1969

There were about forty or forty-five people that we gathered in the center of the village . . . men, women, children . . . babies. . . . Lieutenant Calley . . . started shooting them. And he told me to start shooting. I poured about four clips into the group . . . I fired them on automatic . . . I might have killed ten or fifteen of them. . . . So we started to gather them up, more people . . . we put them in the hootch, and we dropped a hand grenade in there with them . . . they had about seventy or seventy-five people all gathered up. So we threw ours in with them and Lieutenant Calley . . . started pushing them off . . . into the ravine . . . and just started using automatics on them . . . men, women, children . . . and babies. . . . It just seemed like it was the natural thing to do at the time.

> Paul Meadlo,
> Former U.S. Army private, American Division,
> describing the massacre at My Lai, South Vietnam
> Interview on CBS-TV
> November 24, 1969

We should be proud of our country because the American Division rules of engagement are based on Judeo-Christian traditions and are moral, unlike those of the enemy.*

> Lieutenant Colonel James E. Shaw,
> Chief Chaplain, American Division,
> Chulai, South Vietnam
> November 29, 1969

* *Testifying at an unofficial inquiry in December, 1970 in Washington, D.C., into U.S. atrocities in Vietnam, a former Army surgeon, Dr. Gordon Livingston, of Johns Hopkins University, stated that when he was with the 11th Armored Cavalry regiment in Vietnam under Colonel George S. Patton III, Patton asked the chaplain to pray for a big body count of Vietcong. According to Dr. Livingston, the chaplain prayed: "O Lord, give us the wisdom to find the bastards and the strength to pile on."*

Regarding Colonel Patton, Seymour Hersh writes in his book My Lai Four: *"He would exhort his men before combat by telling them, 'I do like to see the arms and legs fly.' He once told his staff, 'The present ratio of 90 percent killing to 10 percent pacification is just about right.' Patton celebrated Christmas in 1968 by sending cards reading: 'From Colonel and Mrs. George S. Patton III—Peace on Earth.' Attached to the cards were color photographs of dismembered Vietcong soldiers stacked in a neat pile."*

Book Two

Hymns of the Military-Industrial Complex

6

A Mighty Fortress
Is Our God

In which, in the name of defending the nation,
the military-industrial complex prospers
while the nation is duped, defrauded and despoiled

May be sung in unison. In majestic style

I look to you not only to protect your country, but to protect your country's purse, to safeguard not only her military strength but her financial stability.

> President Johnson, addressing
> military and civilian officials
> at the Pentagon
> December 11, 1963

Today Defense Department workers in the Pentagon number about 27,000, enough people to fill a fair-sized city. . . . More than half of every tax dollar is spent there.

> Lieutenant Colonel Gene Guerney
> *The Pentagon,* 1964

We will cut our military spending by at least $500 million in the coming fiscal year . . .

Secretary McNamara
Austin, Texas
December 23, 1964

The contractors engaged in this important [defense] effort have pledged a dollar's value for every dollar spent, and this value is being reflected in lower costs to the American people for their national defense.

President Johnson
Washington, D.C.
April 28, 1965

MILITARY SPENDING: ON THE WAY UP AGAIN
Newsweek
May 17, 1965

The May-June rise for aircraft buying was 72%, for shipbuilding, 75%, for missiles, 98%. Missile purchases in the 1966 month show up 40 times higher than those a year earlier.

Business Week
October 29, 1966

JOHNSON TO SEEK $9-BILLION MORE
FOR VIETNAM WAR
New York Times
December 7, 1966

. . . the expansion of defense spending contributed to a significant change in the climate of opinion. The Vietnam build-up virtually assured American businessmen that no economic reverse would occur in the near future.

President Johnson
Economic Report to Congress
January 1967

I don't know of a time in recent history when the military have come to Congress and asked for money for military equipment that they haven't gotten it.

Admiral Hyman Rickover (Ret.)
Testimony before Armed Services Committee
April 18, 1967

BIGGEST ARMS BILL YET

Approved by both House and Senate with only slight differences was the biggest single appropriation bill in the nation's history—69.9 billion dollars for the Defense Department. . . .

Included in the new appropriation bill is approximately 20 billion dollars for the Vietnam war. Odds are that will not be enough.

U.S. News & World Report
September 4, 1967

. . . I sincerely believe any arms race with the Soviet Union would act to our benefit. I believe that we can out-invent, out-research, out-develop, out-engineer and out-produce the U.S.S.R. in any area from sling shots to space weapons, and in so doing become more prosperous while the Soviets become progressively poorer. This is the faith I have in the free enterprise system. . . .

General Curtis LeMay
America Is in Danger, 1968

A Congress which has no trouble raising $80 billions a year for our overgrown military machine . . . cannot find $6 billions in budget cuts without reducing the relative pittance we spend on poverty and urban unrest.

I.F. Stone's Weekly
May 27, 1968

69

According to the [Pentagon] list, more than $9 billion was spent on 66 projects before they were abandoned as unnecessary, unworkable, or useless. Among them were 19 different aircraft projects and 28 different missile systems.

From an article by Saul Friedman,
Washington correspondent for Knight Newspapers,
inserted in *Congressional Record*
March 26, 1969

We now have a military-industrial team with unique resources of experience, engineering talent, management and problem-solving capacities, a team that must be used to help find the answers to complex weapons systems. These answers can be put to good use by our cities and our states, by our schools, by large and small business alike.

Secretary of Defense Clifford
Quoted by Bernard D. Nossiter
Washington Post
December 8, 1968

ARMS FIRMS . . . LEADERS SHOW LITTLE INTEREST
IN APPLYING SKILLS TO DOMESTIC ILLS
Washington Post
December 8, 1968

Its [the defense industry's] selling appeal is defense of the home. This is one of the greatest appeals the politicians have to adjusting the system. If you're the President and you need a control factor in the economy, and you need to sell this factor, you can't sell Harlem and Watts but you can sell self-preservation . . .

Samuel F. Downer, vice-president LTV Aerospace
quoted by Bernard D. Nossiter
Washington Post
December 8, 1968

I consider the Department of Defense to be a Department of Peace.

> President Nixon
> Washington, D.C.
> February 6, 1969

What the military has tried to do for nearly two centuries of American history . . . is, if possible, to prevent wars, minimize the pain of peacetime defense as much as possible, and yet protect the American people so that they can live in peace and freedom as they wish.

> General Wheeler
> Chairman, Joint Chiefs of Staff
> April 11, 1969
> Quoted in *What They Said in 1969*

Deterrence is our primary mission, and peace is our profession. We have a mixed force of bombers and missiles to carry out this mission.

> General Bruce C. Halloway
> Commander in Chief, Strategic Air Command
> Chicago, Illinois, July 29, 1969

America has become a militaristic and aggressive nation. . . . We maintain more than 1,517,000 Americans in uniform overseas in 119 countries. . . . We have an immense and expensive military establishment fueled by a gigantic defense industry. . . . Today the active armed forces contain over 3.4 million men and women. . . .

For far too many senior professional officers, war and combat are an exciting adventure. . . . It is this influential nucleus of aggressive, ambitious professional military leaders who are at the root of America's evolving militarism.

. . . Standing closely behind these leaders, encouraging and

71

prompting them, are the rich and powerful defense industries. . . .
Militarism in America is in full bloom . . .

> General David M. Shoup
> Former Commandant U.S. Marine Corps
> Article in *The Atlantic*
> April 1969

Taken together, the military-industrial team, which protects our national interest against foreign enemies, constitutes at the same time a vital national resource that contributes on an ever-increasing scale to solutions for many of our domestic ills.

> U.S. Air Force Assiocation
> annual policy statement, 1969

When you hear the criticism of the military complex in this country . . . of what we are necessarily doing in the cause of peace and freedom in Vietnam—just remember that history will record that never has a great nation had military forces which were more dedicated and whose activity made a greater contribution to peace than the United States.

> President Nixon
> Aboard U.S.S. *Saratoga,* near
> Norfolk, Virginia, May 17, 1969

. . . Since World War II we have spent roughly 10 times as much on warfare and its attendant requirements as we have on the welfare of our people.

> Senator Fulbright
> Washington, D.C.
> June 4, 1969

A responsible government has a duty to be prudent when it spends the people's money. There is no more justification for

72

wasting money on unnecessary military hardware than there is for wasting it on unwarranted social programs.

President Nixon
Colorado Springs, Colorado
June 4, 1969

According to Senate Majority Leader Mike Mansfield, the U.S. has spent $23 billion on missile systems that either were never deployed or were abandoned. In a paranoid system, waste is a way of life.

. . . If one rationale for building a new weapons system is exposed as nonsense, others spring up to take its place.

. . . Virtually the only people making decisions as to whether new weapons systems are needed, whether they cost too much, and who should make them, are men who directly and personally stand to benefit from big defense budgets.

Richard J. Barnet
The Economy of Death, 1969

It is open season on the armed forces. Military programs are ridiculed as needless if not deliberate waste. The military profession is derided in some of the best circles. Patriotism is considered by some to be a backward, unfashionable fetish of the uneducated and unsophisticated.

President Nixon
Colorado Springs, Colorado
June 4, 1969

The current national debate on the size of the military budget, on the justification of a number of expensive weapons systems and force levels, and on the relative merits of other nonmilitary progress, must not be stifled by anyone, even by the President of the

73

United States. The false, sacred mantle has been lifted from this subject.

Senator William Proxmire
Washington, D.C.
June 5, 1969

The current substitute for serious thought is a cliché about a military-industrial complex. . . .

. . . This I find strangest of all. . . . I cannot imagine that anybody on this committee would take seriously the thought that such great people as General Marshall or Joe Collins or Hoyt Vandenberg or General Bradley or Admiral Forrest Sherman or Admiral Allen Kirk would be engaged in a conspiracy to waste the funds and money of the United States uselessly. And today their counterparts are equally incapable of such action. I should hope that that foolish cliché will be dropped for good.

Dean Acheson, former Secretary of State
Hearings before Joint Subcommittee
on Economy in Government
June 11, 1969

Quite simply the MIC [Military-Industrial Complex] consists of the sprawling Pentagon and its network of defense suppliers and research facilities that together produce America's armed might. During the course of the cold war it has grown into an $80 billion-a-year juggernaut consuming a tenth of the nation's giant-sized gross national product. . . .

Sen. Gaylord Nelson of Wisconsin says: "The whole economy is infiltrated. We are a warfare state."

Newsweek
June 9, 1969

"Thank heavens for the military-industrial complex," said Barry Goldwater of Arizona in a recent Senate statement. "It's ultimate

74

aim is peace in our time, regardless of the aggressive, militaristic image that the left wing is attempting to give it."

Newsweek
June 9, 1969

Senator Goldwater, . . . you put into the record that over 2,000 retired generals, admirals, Navy captains, and Army colonels are working for defense contractors, three times as many as were working for them in 1959.

Senator Proxmire,
Hearing before Joint Subcommittee
on Economy in Government
June 10, 1969

We must do everything in our power to insure that the mental picture Americans have of the Army is that of a winner—an efficient, dynamic, dedicated and socially progressive organization.

General Westmoreland
Quoted in *Newsweek*
June 9, 1969

The cost of developing the F-111 [bomber-fighter plane] was originally estimated at $700 million by General Dynamics and $900 million by military analysts. By 1968, actual development costs had soared to $2 billion. . . .

Many similar experiences of recent years can be cited. . . .

Indeed, in the aerospace industry, source selection competitions [among defense contractors] are often called "bidding and lying" competitions.

Professor Frederick M. Scherer
Consultant for the Federal Council
for Science and Technology,
Hearing before Joint Economic Subcommittee
June 9, 1969

CHAIRMAN PROXMIRE: Mr. Rule, the statement you have just made to Congressman Moorhead—if the Pentagon were honest with the contractor and the contractor honest with the Pentagon, and the Pentagon honest with Congress, and the Congress honest with itself, we might scrub some of these weapons systems—is one of the most revealing and significant statements that has been made at these whole hearings. . . .

Are we being lied to? Is that what you are telling us?

GORDON W. RULE (Director, Procurement Control and Clearance, Office of Navy Materiel): That word "lied" and that word "honest" are your words, not mine.

CHAIRMAN PROXMIRE: It is a soft lie, a white lie; it is a nice lie, but it is a lie. . . . We are not being told the truth.

MR. RULE: The Government, the Department of Defense, the service involved, and the contractor, they know that it is going to cost more. And if that is being dishonest—

CHAIRMAN PROXMIRE: Of course, it is being dishonest, if they know it, and if they say it is going to cost less, that is being dishonest. That is a deception for the Congress and the taxpayer. And it is just as wrong as it can be.

MR. RULE: I think it is wrong, but I think it would only be disingenuous.

> Hearing before Joint Economic Subcommittee
> June 10, 1969

Secretary Laird has charged his entire management team with the task of insuring the integrity of Department of Defense fund requests in the first instance and then the spending of these funds under conditions of maximum efficiency.

> Assistant Secretary of Defense Barry J. Shillito
> Hearing before Joint Economic Subcommittee
> June 11, 1969

I don't see anything improper in the relationship between the military and industry. . . . There are tens of thousands of companies doing defense work. . . . And it is all done through the free-enterprise system: The competition is severe, the risks great, the profits generally lower than in commercial practice.

> Roger Lewis
> President and Chairman of
> the Board, General Dynamics
> Quoted in *Look* magazine
> August 26, 1969

I do not want to see this nation spend one dollar more on defense than is absolutely necessary. . . .

> Vice President Agnew
> New Orleans, Louisiana
> October 9, 1969

WASHINGTON—Major United States weapons systems are costing at least $20 billion more than original estimates—and no man knows the total number of systems being acquired or their costs, Congress was told yesterday.

> Associated Press
> *San Francisco Chronicle*
> December 30, 1969

We maintain our strength but we maintain it for peace.

> President Nixon
> Quoted in *The American Legion Magazine*
> December 1969

. . . the final challenge which confronts our nation as we move into the '70's [is] the challenge of lowered defense spending. . . . The real danger lies in the attempt to cut defense programs even more.

> Admiral Thomas H. Moorer
> Chairman, Joint Chiefs of Staff
> Detroit, Michigan
> November 9, 1970

From 1946 to 1969, the United States Government spent over $1,000 billion on the military. . . .

. . . the fiscal 1970 budget plan of the Department of Defense—$83 *billion*—exceeds the gross national product . . . of entire nations. . . .

. . . military activity has come to permeate many aspects of American society . . . with the result that the whole society begins to take on something of the character of a "garrison society."

> Seymour Melman
> *Pentagon Capitalism—*
> *The Political Economy of War, 1970*°

U.S. [FOREIGN] MILITARY ASSISTANCE FOR 1970 IS PUT AT 8 TIMES THE FIGURE IN THE BUDGET
New York Times
January 7, 1971

PENTAGON SPENDING . . . TO HEAD UPWARD
New York Times
January 10, 1971

° *"By fiscal year 1971," wrote Professor Melman in an article in the* New York Times *on November 3, 1970, "the Federal budget used 64.8 percent of tax dollars to pay for wars, past and present."*

7

𝕸𝖞 𝕱𝖆𝖎𝖙𝖍 𝕷𝖔𝖔𝖐𝖘 𝖀𝖕 𝖙𝖔 𝕿𝖍𝖊𝖊

*In which, while the F-111 fighter-bomber
is lauded as the best of all planes,
it has difficulty keeping in the air*

Brightly

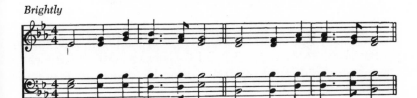

After a stormy birth, which has been very much on my mind for many months, the F-111 is recognized for what it is: a truly enormous advance in the art of military aircraft.

The plane is the greatest single step forward in combat aircraft in several decades.

> Secretary of Defense McNamara
> Fort Worth, Texas
> October 15, 1964

WASHINGTON, Dec. 22 (AP)—Yesterday's first test flight of the F-111 at Forth Worth was described by the Pentagon as a spectacular success.

> *New York Times*
> December 23, 1964

FLIGHT TESTS STIR WORRY OVER F-111
PIVOT-WING PLANE BESET BY TECHNICAL TROUBLES
New York Times
March 10, 1965

Senator McClellan asked the [general] accounting office to investigate reports that the unit cost of the TFX, now in production as the F-111, had almost doubled since 1963. . . .
New York Times
August 17, 1966

WASHINGTON, Sept. 9 (UPI)—The Defense Department, answering critics of the F-111 warplane, told Congress today . . . [It] will be superior in its class to any other tactical weapons system in the world."
New York Times
September 10, 1966

DELAY IN F-111 SEEN AS RESULT OF CRASH
New York Times
January 21, 1967

2 DIE IN LONG ISLAND CRASH OF F-111B TEST JET
New York Times
April 22, 1967

GENERAL DYNAMICS GETS F-111 AWARD WORTH $1.8 BILLION
New York Times
May 11, 1967

WASHINGTON, June 1 (AP)— . . . The deputy chief for air [Vice Admiral T. F. Connolly] describes the controversial F-111B aircraft as an easy plane to fly, with outstanding low-speed qualities, and predicts it will be an impressive airplane.

New York Times
June 2, 1967

NEW TROUBLES WITH F-111 PLANE
DELAY COMBAT TESTS IN VIETNAM
New York Times
August 11, 1967

WASHINGTON, Sept. 13—Significant new shortcomings of the F-111 swing-wing airplane were disclosed here today.

Richard Witkin
New York Times
September 14, 1967

F-111A DEVELOPS FIRE IN TAIL
DURING NEVADA TEST FLIGHTS
New York Times
September 23, 1967

No matter what you read in the newspapers, [the F-111] does fly. . . .

It's certainly the most advanced aircraft right now, I suspect, in the whole world.

General G.P. Disosway
Commander, Air Force Tactical Air Command
Las Vegas, Nevada
September 24, 1967

2 ESCAPE AS F-111A CRASHES IN TEXAS
New York Times
October 20, 1967

F-111 CRASHES ON TRAINING FLIGHT
NEAR EDWARDS AIR FORCE BASE
New York Times
January 3, 1968

WASHINGTON, March 14 (AP)— . . . Secretary of the Navy Paul R. Ignatius said that most of the deficiencies in the controversial plane had been corrected . . . [He] urged the [Senate Armed Services] Committee to approve funds for 30 production models for which funds are sought in the new defense budget.

New York Times
March 15, 1968

FIRST F-111 JET LOST AND
NORTH VIETNAM REPORTS DOWNING IT
New York Times
March 29, 1968

SECOND F-111 JET FIGHTER
DOWN IN SOUTHEAST ASIA
New York Times
March 31, 1968

DEFENSE AIDE CONFIRMS F-111 IS GROUNDED
New York Times
April 2, 1968

WASHINGTON, April 15 (UPI)—The Air Force has reenacted the circumstances that led to the crash of a controversial F-111 fighter-bomber in Thailand last month and believes it has eliminated the trouble, informed sources said today.

New York Times
April 16, 1968

BANGKOK, Thailand, April 21 (UPI)—The Secretary of the Air Force, Harold Brown, concluded a three-day tour of United States bases in Thailand today and said he was satisfied with the controversial F-111A fighter-bomber.

New York Times
April 22, 1968

THIRD F-111 CRASHES, THAILAND,
APPARENTLY BECAUSE OF MECHANICAL FAILURE
New York Times
April 25, 1968

CHICAGO, April 24—Lagging profits, a corporate image, the sagging price of stock and . . . the F-111 jet fighter were the chief matters of concern today at the annual stockholders meeting of the General Dynamics Corporation. . . .

"The situation in connection with the F-111 is somewhat different," Mr. Lewis [president and chairman of General Dynamics] said. "There is no question of anticipated losses. The question is how much profit to book in a given year."

Robert Wright
New York Times
April 25, 1968

F-111 CRASH LANDS AT AIR FORCE SHOW
New York Times
May 19, 1968

Development of the F-111 over the last five years . . . [has] cost the nation approximately $8 billion.

New York Times
August 18, 1968

NAVY F-111 CRASHES INTO OCEAN WITH 2
New York Times
September 12, 1968

The Air Force ordered a temporary halt to all F-111 flights yesterday after a crash Monday at a base in Las Vegas. . . . Monday's crash was the second this month and the 11th since the plane began flying.

Richard Witkin
New York Times
September 25, 1968

WASHINGTON, Oct. 25— . . . Conceding that he has before him proposals to cut back the F-111 aircraft program [Secretary of Defense] Clifford said it was the opinion of his office and of the Air Force that the plane was an excellent one. The Defense Secretary complained that there had been what he regarded as "overemphasis" on the early difficulties of the F-111, ten of which have crashed in this country and Southeast Asia.

William Beecher
New York Times
October 26, 1968

The F-111 in a Nixon Administration will be made into one of the foundations of our air supremacy.

Richard M. Nixon
El Paso, Texas
November 2, 1968

MISSING F-111A IS HUNTED
IN UTAH AND NEVADA WILDS
New York Times
February 14, 1969

F-111 ENCOUNTERS ANOTHER "WING BOX" PROBLEM
AS CRACK DEVELOPS
New York Times
February 18, 1969

NELLIS A.F.B., Nev., March 4 (UPI)—An F-111A fighter-bomber crashed today. . . . The plane was the 2nd F-111A to crash in less than three weeks and the 13th to crash since the flight test program began.

> *New York Times*
> March 5, 1969

The F-111 is a fantastic airplane. . . . [It] not only does its thing. . . . It does it better than any other airplane in the Air Force.

> Major Thomas Wheeler, Jr.
> Quoted in *The Airman*
> August 1969

The Senate Permanent Subcommittee on Investigations issued a report in Washington yesterday calling the multibillion-dollar F-111 fighter-bomber program a "fiscal blunder of the worst magnitude."

Of the 500 [planes] to be built, the subcommittee said, fewer than 100 will "come reasonably close" to performing as originally intended. . . .

Among the contentions the report made were the following:

Roswell L. Gilpatrick, Deputy Secretary of Defense under Mr. McNamara, "was guilty of a flagrant conflict of interest" in the awarding of the F-111 airframe contract to the General Dynamics Corporation. He was "top level policy counselor" to the company for two and a half years before going to the Pentagon. . . .

Testimony given by [Secretary of Defense] McNamara was termed at various points "obviously intentionally deceptive," . . . and "an obvious and artful attempt to avoid telling the truth.

> Richard Witkin
> *New York Times*
> December 19, 1970

85

8

Ride On! Ride On in Majesty!

*In which tanks hailed
as the most advanced and deadly of all armored vehicles
have a tendency to blow themselves up*

Confidently

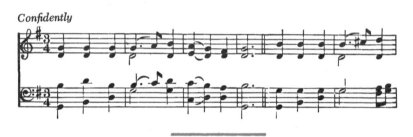

The General Sheridan Weapon System, with the Shillegah [anti-tank missile], will provide the army with a major advancement in tanklike weapon systems and a significant improvement in fire power. . . .

> Colonel Paul A. Simpson
> Sheridan Project Manager
> U.S. Weapons Command
> March 29, 1966

. . . American tank experts who are close to the program insist that . . . the MBT-70 [Main Battle Tank] will be the fastest, deadliest and most advanced armored combat vehicle ever devised and promises the allies a decided edge over Soviet armor.*

William Beecher
New York Times
October 9, 1967

A futuristic tank with . . . a gun capable of firing missiles and artillery shells is to be unveiled . . . in the United States and Germany after four years of joint development by the two countries.

Called the Main Battle Tank . . . , the armored vehicle has fallen a year behind production schedule and is experiencing serious problems with its weapons system. . . .

. . . In a few instances premature explosions [inside the tank's turret] have occurred . . .

William Beecher
New York Times
October 9, 1967

I really don't know what the Russians have, but I'd like to place a bet for a month's pay that this is better.

Major General Edwin H. Burba
top U.S. officer on the American-German team
developing Main Battle Tank
October 9, 1967

* *The Main Battle Tank (MBT-70) and the General Sheridan Weapon System or Sheridan, an armored reconnaissance assault vehicle, were both designed to use the same new turret system with a gun to fire missiles as well as conventional shells. However, as was later disclosed at hearings of the House Armed Services Committee, there was one problem with the turret system. The Army could find no ammunition that functioned properly in it.*

Despite this disconcerting fact, the Army ordered full-scale production of the Sheridan. In a confidential memorandum on April 4, 1966, Major General William B. Bunker of the Army Materiel Command explained to his associates that delaying production because of the faulty ammunition "would have both adverse political and budgetary impacts."

BONN, Oct. 9—The West German Defense Ministry unveiled today . . . a prototype of the Main Battle Tank of the 1970's. . . .

After thirty minutes of maneuverability test, smoke began pouring out of the turret. The three-man crew jumped out uninjured and called for fire extinguishers. . . . The tank could not be used for the rest of the demonstration. . . .

> Philip Shabecoff
> *New York Times*
> October 10, 1967

Although the cost of the [MBT-70] program has risen substantially above the original estimates, it is believed that the tank will meet or surpass nearly all of its performance objectives.

> Secretary of Defense McNamara
> Defense Posture Statement
> January, 1968

West Germany is going to give up research on the MBT-70. . . . The American defense organization has . . . spent a fortune on wining and dining of foreign defense experts in an attempt to sell this tank. The West Germans want to get out because they can see no future market for the tank in Western Europe.

> *Atlanta Journal*
> February 14, 1969

"If allowance is made for the initial two years when we were feeling our way, then the MBT-70 program can be considered on schedule," one [Defense Department] official told this magazine.

> *Aerospace Technology*
> February 26, 1968

The Army purchased Sheridan weapons, E-1 tank turret systems, and E-2 tanks, all incorporating the combination gun missile launcher, even though no acceptable ammunition was available for this gun launcher. . . . Furthermore, mass production of the Sheridan was permitted to continue. . . . As a matter of fact, fully acceptable ammunition still has not been developed.

Elmer B. Staats,
U.S. Comptroller General
Hearing before House Armed Services Subcommittee
May 13, 1969

My information is that at the present time we spent something like $2.3 billion of the taxpayers' money to develop a weapons system. This system is today nonoperative, because of the fact that we've got a lot of tanks sitting out on a parking lot with no ammunition to fire out of them. And I think the taxpayers of this country . . . are justifiably concerned about how the U.S. Army can waste $2 billion of the taxpayers' money in developing a weapon that 10 years later isn't worth a darn.

Representative Samuel S. Stratton
Washington, D.C.
March 20, 1969

Army officials . . . say that two squadrons of Sheridans, about 54 in all, have been operating successfully in Vietnam since February. . . . These two squadrons were sent on an experimental basis, but the results have been so favorable that the Army has now decided to begin deploying hundreds of Sheridans in Vietnam.

Neil Sheehan
New York Times
May 15; 1969

The Sheridan was sent to Vietnam, Lieutenant General A. W. Betts, chief of Army research and development said, because it was "urgent" to use it there and worth the "calculated technical risks." Betts said two weeks ago that the Sheridan had "clearly proved their combat worth, in spite of the technical bugs."

Times-Post Service
San Francisco Chronicle
June 17, 1969

An Army armored vehicle sent into combat . . . has experienced breakdowns and deficiencies that have jeopardized United States troops in combat, according to a secret Pentagon report. . . .

The report listed 15 major equipment failures, 125 electronic circuit failures, 41 weapon misfires, 140 ammunition ruptures, 25 engine replacements . . . and persistent failure of the recoil mechanism of the Sheridan's 152 mm. gun.

Times-Post Service
San Francisco Chronicle
June 17, 1969

Just announced: 171 new Sheridans are to be shipped to Vietnam.

The Nation
July 7, 1969

It is a fine vehicle for Vietnam.

Colonel Merritte W. Ireland,
commander of Army unit
that battle-tested Sheridans,
July 10, 1969

WASHINGTON, July 9—The United States Army's embattled Sheridan and M-60 tank systems came under renewed attack today in a congressional report . . . prepared by the Investigations Subcommittee of the House Armed Services Committee. The compilation of the project's 10 year history alleges the following:

. . . "Misleading reports and unwarranted overconfidence by Army developers" influenced the crucial decisions.

The subcommittee accused Army representatives of a "total lack of candor" in parts of their testimony.

New York Times
July 10, 1969

The Army insists that problems with the Sheridan—more specifically its weapons—now are solved.

Business Week
August 9, 1969

REPRESENTATIVE SAMUEL S. STRATTON: Mr. Chairman, I would like just to have the record show this is a vehicle on which well over a billion dollars was spent in 10 years of development, and the Army is phasing it out after a couple of years of production.

REPRESENTATIVE PHILIP J. PHILBIN: The record may so show . . .

Hearing before House
Armed Services Subcommittee
March 25, 1970

9

Ten Thousand Times
Ten Thousand

*In which a purported saving by the Defense Department
costs taxpayers billions of dollars, and the price
of telling the truth is dismissal from the Pentagon*

Joyfully

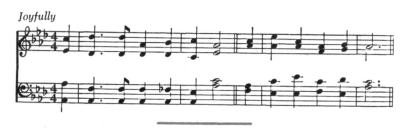

WASHINGTON, Sept. 30 (UPI)—The Government awarded a $2
billion contract to the Lockheed Aircraft Corporation, to build a
fleet of giant transport planes, each capable of carrying 600 armed
soldiers.

The plane, to be known as the C-5A, would be the largest jet
transport ever built. . . .

Despite the initial outlay, Defense Secretary Robert S. McNamara is convinced the long-term cost of operation . . . will be
less than that for the current largest military transport. . . . He
has estimated that the cost reduction will amount to as much as
30 or 40 percent.

New York Times
October 1, 1965

JOINT PANEL TOLD OF RISE IN C-5A COST

WASHINGTON, Nov. 13 (UPI)—An Air Force spokesman conceded today that the Pentagon might end up paying the Lockheed Aircraft Corporation double the original contract estimate for building 115 C-5A military cargo jets.

This disclosure was made by A. E. Fitzgerald, Air Force Deputy for management systems. He testified at a hearing of Congressional Joint Economic Committee.

> *New York Times*
> November 11, 1968

PENTAGON TO BUY MORE CARGO JETS
C-5A's WILL BE PURCHASED
DESPITE COST INVESTIGATION

. . . The Pentagon action came hours before the Joint Economic Committee resumed its investigation into what its Chairman, Senator William Proxmire, described as "the shocking cost escalation" of the C-5A jet.

"This is the most fantastic overrun I've ever heard of," the Wisconsin Democrat said.

> Marjorie Hunter
> *New York Times*
> January 17, 1969

CHAIRMAN PROXMIRE: . . . I would like to ask you a few questions concerning . . . the testimony before this committee last November of Mr. A. E. Fitzgerald, an Air Force official. Mr. Fitzgerald was instructed not to provide a written statement for the subcommittee . . . even though we requested one. Did you have anything to do with the decision to instruct the witness not to give a written statement?

ASSISTANT SECRETARY OF THE AIR FORCE ROBERT H. CHARLES: Not directly. . . .

93

CHAIRMAN PROXMIRE: Well, there was also some effort made in the Defense Department to prevent Mr. Fitzgerald from testifying at all. . . . Now, Mr. Charles, I would like to ask you, do you know whether any further action is planned or contemplated against Mr. Fitzgerald?

MR. CHARLES: I not only know of no further action that is planned against him, I know of none that has been taken against him.

Hearing before Joint
Economic Subcommittee
January 16, 1969

Senator Proxmire . . . made public a memorandum, prepared by Air Force Secretary Harold Brown earlier this month . . . listing ways in which Mr. Fitzgerald might be dismissed. . . . The Air Force action, Senator Proxmire charged, "is the most shocking example of retaliation against a public servant I have seen in the 11 years I have been in the Senate."

Marjorie Hunter
New York Times
January 17, 1969

WASHINGTON, April 30— . . . Details of the enormous increase in the cost of developing the [C-5A] aircraft and of the Air Force's doctoring of documents to protect Lockheed Aircraft Corporation, the company holding the C-5A contract, were made public yesterday in hearings before the House Government Operations Subcommittee on Military Operations.

. . . Col. Kenneth N. Beckman, the officer in charge of the C-5A contract, testified that his civilian superiors—Robert H. Charles, Assistant Secretary of the Air Force . . . and Robert N.

Anthony, the former Defense Department Controller—had agreed to suppress data on the ground that disclosure might jeopardize Lockheed's position on the stock market.

David E. Rosenbaum
New York Times
May 1, 1969

MARIETTA, Ga., May 1 (UPI)—The chairman of the board of the Lockheed Aircraft Corporation, maker of the C-5A jet transport, today blamed "incomplete and inaccurate" reporting of a Congressional hearing for the latest furor over the cost of the world's largest plane.

New York Times
May 2, 1969

I think we have in the C-5A contract the best contract ever entered into by the Air Force. I think it is a shame and a disservice to the Air Force and to sound procurement practices, that it has been unfairly criticized.

Assistant Secretary of the Air Force Charles
Quoted in *Aviation Week*
May 12, 1969

It was originally estimated that the cost of these [C-5A] planes would be $2.9 billion, but it subsequently became clear to Pentagon officials that the actual cost would exceed $5.9 billion. Yet, according to the testimony of an Air Force officer before the House Operations Committee, that information was concealed by doctoring the records with the approval of civilian officials in the Pentagon.

Editorial
New York Times
May 12, 1969

Said [Secretary of Defense] Laird: "I don't want to prejudge the case," while the Air Force is investigating, but "it is important to restore the credibility of the Pentagon."

Newsweek
May 12, 1969

I want to assure this subcommittee, the Congress, and the American people that all of the officials and employees of the Department of Defense—and particularly those who play a role in managing its affairs—are dedicated to rooting out waste and inefficiency wherever and whenever they appear. This is a never-ending task. . . .

We welcome . . . constructive suggestions from this and other Committees of the Congress.

Assistant Secretary of Defense Barry J. Shillito
Hearings before Joint Economic Subcommittee
June 11, 1969

The Pentagon yesterday fired A. Ernest Fitzgerald, the Air Force efficiency expert who first disclosed the $2 billion cost overrun on the C-5A. . . .

Sen. William Proxmire . . . called the firing a "reprisal." . . . Proxmire declared: "The firing of A. E. Fitzgerald is a clear message from the Pentagon to its employees. That message is, 'Do not try to reduce costs; do not aim towards efficiency; do not attempt to achieve economy in government; if you do, you will be isolated and fired.' "

Bernard D. Nossiter
Washington Post
November 5, 1969

A brief [Air Force] announcement said that A. E. Fitzgerald's position in the Pentagon . . . was being eliminated as a part of the Defense Department's effort to save money.

New York Times
November 5, 1969

CHAIRMAN PROXMIRE: Can you tell us, Secretary Seamans, whom you consulted with prior to making your decision to fire Fitzgerald? Did you talk the matter over with Mr. Fitzgerald?

SECRETARY OF THE AIR FORCE ROBERT C. SEAMANS, JR.: I did not decide to fire Mr. Fitzgerald.

CHAIRMAN PROXMIRE: Well, dismiss Mr. Fitzgerald, if you prefer that word.

SECRETARY SEAMANS: I prefer to use the correct term, which is to abolish his job.*

> Hearing before Joint
> Economic Subcommittee
> November 18, 1969

* *A few days after Ernest Fitzgerald's job was "abolished" in the name of "saving money," the Air Force hired a new man to replace him at a considerably higher salary. The man's name was John Dyment, and, coincidentally enough, he had been previously employed by Arthur Young & Company, the accounting firm for Lockheed Aircraft, the firm that built the C-5A. Noteworthy was the fact that Arthur Young & Company was co-defendant with Lockheed in a suit charging that the two firms cheated Lockheed stockholders by concealing from them the truth about the cost overruns on the C-5A.*

The new appointment caused such a furor in Congress that the Air Force soon canceled Dyment's contract.

10

While Shepherds Watched Their Flocks by Night

*In which, despite protestations of innocence
by the Pentagon, it is established that
thousands of dead sheep did not commit suicide*

With tender feeling

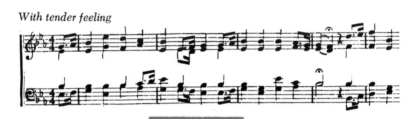

WASHINGTON—Perhaps 5,000 sheep have sickened and died in the past week in Western Utah in a place called Skull Valley, 20 or 30 miles from the Army's main site for field-testing chemical and biological weapons. That center, the Army's Dugway Proving Grounds site, "definitely is not responsible," a Dugway spokesman said yesterday. "Our scientists have ruled out [as a cause of the sheep deaths] programs which are part of our mission."

Time-Post Service
San Francisco Chronicle
March 21, 1968

When we first found out about it, we checked and found we hadn't been running any tests that could have caused this.

Army Public Relations Officer
at Dugway Proving Grounds
Quoted in *Salt Lake Tribune*
March 21, 1968

WILLOW SPRINGS, Utah, March 21— . . . Tonight the Washington office of Senator Frank E. Moss, Utah Democrat, said that Senator Moss had been told by the Army Testing Command that : . . on March 13, two days before the sheep began collapsing and dying . . . 320 gallons of a "persistent gas" was sprayed from an airplane.

The tests were from 15 to 27 miles from the place where the sheep were grazing.*

Wallace Turner
New York Times
March 22, 1968

SALT LAKE CITY, March 23 (AP)—The head of a special investigating team said today that "we are as positive as medical science can ever be" that nerve gas tests conducted at the Army's top-secret Dugway Proving Grounds had killed 6400 sheep in Western Utah's Skull Valley.

Dr. D. A. Osguthorpe said that he believed that "sufficient

---

* *In his book,* The Ultimate Folly, *Congressman Richard D. McCarthy later related: "When the sheep began toppling over, ranchers summoned Dr. D. Avaron Osguthorpe, a veterinarian. He soon conjectured that the writhing sheep had been affected by nerve gas and contacted [Dugway] officers. . . . They informed him that there had been no outdoor nerve gas tests since the preceding year. . . ."*

"The first admission that nerve gas testing actually had taken place on March 13, 1968, came inadvertently from the Pentagon eight days after the test. The Department of Defense sent Senator Frank E. Moss a letter describing the test. An aide to the Senator . . . ignored or was unaware of the fact that the Pentagon regarded the letter as private and released it to the press."

99

tests" had been made to link the deaths with Army operations. "We're very lucky no people were killed," he added.

New York Times
March 24, 1968

. . . An Army spokesman said that the military investigation was continuing, and that "no definite cause of death" had been established.

New York Times
March 24, 1968

We do not have any evidence to tell us the actual chemical compound or to help us pinpoint the source and how it got to the sheep and not to humans or to other animals.

General William S. Stone,
officer in charge of Army investigation at Dugway
March 25, 1968

SALT LAKE CITY, March 24 (AP)—Had the Army admitted earlier that it was testing lethal nerve gas in Skull Valley, many of the 6,400 sheep that died could have been saved, a Utah veterinarian charged today.

The veterinarian, Mr. Mar Fawcett, said that many sheep had died because the Army waited several days before admitting making the tests at Dugway Proving Grounds. . . .

"I'm sure if we had known about the testing and had an antidote many of the sheep could have been saved," Dr. Fawcett said.

New York Times
March 25, 1968

Dr. Mortimer Rothenberg . . . who is scientific director at Dugway, said that the sheep symptoms were "completely atypical from what one would anticipate from nerve gas."

- *New York Times*
March 25, 1968

None of the nerve agent which was released from the airplane on March 13 has been discovered in the soil, water or forage of the area where the sheep died.

General William S. Stone
Quoted in statement from Senator Moss's office
March 29, 1968

It would be speculative to fix a specific cause of the death of the sheep.

Lieutenant Colonel William L. Black,
Dugway's executive officer Quoted in *Newsweek*
April 1, 1968

Chemists of NCDC have isolated an identical compound from snow water and grass from White Rock area and from liver, blood and stomach contents of dead sheep from the same area. . . . Compound has been shown identical to test agent supplied by Dr. K. M. Brauner, Dugway, April 4, 1968.

Excerpt from telegram from
National Communicable Disease Center, Atlanta,
Georgia, to Dr. G.D.C. Thompson, Director of
Utah Division of Health
April 12, 1968

WASHINGTON, April 18 (UPI)—The Army conceded today that an unexpected shift in the wind could have carried nerve gas being tested in the Utah desert into an area where about 6,400 sheep mysteriously died.

New York Times
April 19, 1968

After first denying any possible connection with the deaths, the Army has gradually admitted more and more until now they have said everything but the word "guilty." . . .

On April 10 . . . I advised the sheep owners to begin filing claims for reimbursement. The Army has held a meeting with the claimants. . . .

Senator Moss
Article in
Utah Wool Grower
June 1968

WASHINGTON, Dec. 20 (AP)— . . . The Army has said investigations failed to turn up any conclusive evidence that the sheep died because of the gas. However, it has paid a claim of more than $376,000 for the loss of the sheep.

New York Times
December 21, 1968

WASHINGTON, May 21—Under Congressional prodding, the Army admitted for the first time today that its nerve gas killed 6,000 sheep in Utah more than 14 months ago.

The admission was wrung from three Army officials, a shred at a time, during half a day of hard and angry questioning by members of the House Subcommittee on Conservational and National Resources. . . .

The Army spokesmen confirmed, after much verbal jousting, that the public information officer at Dugway had not told the truth when he told reporters last March that Dugway had done no testing that could have caused the sheep to die.

Roy Reed
New York Times
May 22, 1969

The American public are getting fed to the teeth with attempts to deceive them—by the military or anyone else.

Editorial
New York Times
May 23, 1969

11

Tell Me the Old, Old Story

*In which a military chorus offers selections
based on the ancient theme of the Red Menace*

With solemnity

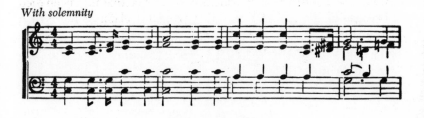

CHAIRMAN GEORGE H. MAHON: You were talking about the Russians being able to do this and that. As a result of this philosophy of what the Russians could do, a few years ago we developed the bomber gap, and later we were told there was no bomber gap.

As a result of this same reasoning as to what the Russians could do, we developed the missile gap. . . . Now we come along later and everyone says there never was a missile gap.

Now, are you by this testimony opening up a so-called megatonnage gap which will never occur and which will be just as phony as the bomber and missile gap?

GENERAL CURTIS LEMAY: This is entirely possible, Mr. Chairman.
Defense Budget hearings before
House Subcommittee on Defense Appropriations,
released April 14, 1964

. . . the military aspects of the Communist threat represent just one phase of the most insidious and gigantic plot in history. There are the economic, technological, ideological and other phases, all designed for one objective only . . . the accomplishment of the ultimate Communist goal of total world domination.

> General Thomas S. Power
> Former Commander, Strategic Air Command
> *Design For Survival*, 1965

Red China under its present leadership seems to me at this writing to be practically a hopeless case. Naked force seems to be the only logic which the leadership of that unfortunate nation can comprehend. . . .

> General Nathan F. Twining
> Former Chairman, Joint Chiefs of Staff
> *Neither Liberty Nor Safety*, 1966

We should give priority to the prevention of subversive insurgency. . . . The next question is, where do you look for symptoms of subversive insurgency? The answer is that they are found in virtually every emerging country in the world.

> General Maxwell Taylor
> Former Chief of Staff, U.S. Army
> American Foreign Service Association luncheon
> March 31, 1966

The Communists' design over the years has been clearly to break down and destroy order with the intent of building the totalitarianism of its oligarchy on the ruins and debris of the past. . . . Today, the military forces of the free world . . . are built toward the purpose of containing violence.

> General C. H. Bonesteel, III
> Essay in *Issues of National
> Security in the 1970's*, 1967

Communists emerged shortly after World War I and have been relentlessly at work ever since attempting to gain influence and power [in Latin America] by eroding American influence and depriving countries of American cooperation. . . . The Communists are bent on destroying these evolving societies. . . .

> General Robert W. Porter, Jr.
> Commander in Chief, U.S. Southern Command
> New York City, New York
> March 26, 1968

. . . it is necessary to understand that Vietnam is part of a much larger and much longer war—a war between communism and the Free World. . . . Although the war has many facets, it has but one objective: Communist control of the entire world.

> General Curtis LeMay
> *American Is in Danger,* 1968

Let us . . . look at some of the key conditions throughout the world which warn us of the problems we face as we go forward.

Foremost is the growing threat of Russia. This threat overshadows all others in terms of immediate risk to our national security. . . .

It is a matter of grave concern that the pendulum of superiority is moving in favor of the Soviet Union.

> Admiral Thomas H. Moorer
> Chairman, Joint Chiefs of Staff
> Detroit, Michigan
> November 9, 1970

The American people have lived with fears of a Soviet attack for some quarter of a century, ever since World War II, and have expended a thousand billion dollars on defense in recognition of this possible danger. These gigantic expenditures have been detrimental to many other plans, programs and policies which now also appear vitally important to the security and well-being of this Nation. The American people now know that many billions of these dollars spent on defense have been wasted.*

Report signed by
Senators Stuart Symington, Stephen M. Young
and Daniel K. Inouye
of the Armed Services Committee
Quoted in *I.F. Stone's Weekly*,
July 28, 1969

---

* *Commenting on this report, I. F. Stone wrote: "The truth is that we have spent a trillion dollars since World War II on a gigantic hoax. The U.S. emerged from World War II, as from World War I, virtually unscathed, enormously enriched and—with the atom bomb—immeasurably more powerful than any nation on the earth had ever been. The notion that it was in danger of attack from a devastated Soviet Union with 25 million war dead, a generation behind it in industrial development, was a wicked fantasy. But this myth has been the mainstay of the military and the war machine."*

Book Three

Hymns of the Promised Land

12

Throw Out the Lifeline

*In which, while prosperity is proclaimed,
poverty abounds and the economy wavers*

With quiet confidence

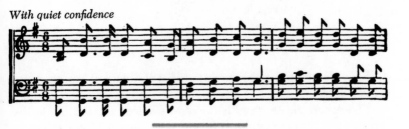

This Administration, here and now, declares unconditional war
on poverty in America . . . wherever it exists . . . in city slums
and small towns, in sharecropper shacks or migrant-worker camps,
on Indian reservations, among whites as well as Negroes, among
the young as well as the aged. . . .

        President Johnson
        State of the Union Message
        January 8, 1964

For the first time in America's history, poverty is on the run. . . .

        President Johnson
        Washington, D.C.
        April 17, 1964

ST. LOUIS, Nov. 15—A national authority on combatting poverty said today that a minimum of $100 billion in the next 10 years was required to cope with the problems of the economically deprived.

. . . Michael Harrington said that "the present program is going to abolish very little poverty." . . . Mr. Harrington, a consultant to Sargent Shriver, head of the Office for Economic Opportunity, is the author of the widely known book, *The Other America; Poverty in the United States.* . . .

> Irving Spiegel
> *New York Times*
> November 16, 1964

I am pleased to be able to report that the state of our economy is excellent. . . .

The American economy is the most efficient and flexible in the world. . . . as our standards for the performance of our economy have risen, so has our ability to cope with our own economic problems.

> President Johnson
> Washington, D.C.
> January 28, 1965

The wealthiest nation in the world has been unable to rally the resources to raise one fifth of its own people from poverty. . . .

The price of building colossal military power and endlessly adding to it has been the depletion of American society. . . . The contradiction between guns and butter is now real and measurable.

> Seymour Melman
> *Our Depleted Society,* 1965

The new budget shows that the main concern of the government is still war; the main beneficiary of its vast expenditures, still the military bureaucracy and its Siamese twin, the armaments industry. . . . At one end of the scale, more than $50 billions for the war machine, 50% of the administrative budget. At the other end of the scale, $1.3 billion for that purely metaphorical "war on poverty." . . .

I.F. Stone's Weekly
February 2, 1965

A year ago I reported that we were "in the midst of the greatest upsurge of economic well-being in the history of the nation." That upsurge, now about to enter its sixth year, continues without letup. . . .

Today, across the Atlantic and around the world one hears once again of "the American economic miracle." . . .

We have again shown the world what free men and a free economy can achieve.

President Johnson
Economic Report to Congress
January 1, 1966

Our country is big enough to support a war in Vietnam and a successful war on poverty at home.

Sargent Shriver,
Director Office of Economic Opportunity
Quoted in *Newsweek*
January 3, 1966

There is a kind of madness in the facile assumption that we can raise the many billions of dollars necessary to rebuild our schools and cities and public transport and eliminate the pollution of air and water while also spending tens of billions to finance an "open-ended" war in Asia . . .

Senator Fulbright
University of Connecticut
March 22, 1966

In summary of the economic picture, Gardner W. Ackley, Chairman of the Council of Economic Advisers, emphasized the gains that have been made in every aspect of the economy in the past two and a half years, which he characterized as having been "spectacularly larger than in the previous decade."

Eileen Shanahan
New York Times
August 12, 1966

SENATE APPROVES ANTIPOVERTY BILL; $746-MILLION CUT
New York Times
October 5, 1966

RISE IN WAR COST REACHES A PEAK
INCREASE FOR QUARTER PUTS DEFENSE SPENDING
AT RATE OF $60 BILLION A YEAR
New York Times
October 5, 1966

Among Administration economists the big news is that the economy's brief touch with recession is ending.

Wall Street Journal
June 26, 1967

RISING COSTS OF WAR THREATEN ECONOMY
Journal of Commerce
September 29, 1967

A strange thing is being discovered: Wages keep going up, yet most workers are no better off than a year or two ago. . . . The typical wage earner is on a treadmill, getting nowhere.

U.S. News & World Report
January 1, 1968

He [Secretary of Defense McNamara] said he felt we could have another war like Vietnam over there and we could handle all of the domestic programs in this country, and at the same time we did both of these things—if we had the will and the determination—we could handle the problems of less fortunate people all over the world.

> Senator Stuart Symington,
> paraphrasing unpublished testimony of Secretary
> McNamara before Senate Foreign Relations
> Committee, Quoted in *New Republic*
> April 6, 1968

At least ten million Americans are victims of hunger. . . .
Whatever happened to President Johnson's commitments to wage all-out war on poverty and hunger?*

> Editorial
> *New York Times*
> April 28, 1968

It's an amazing paradox that the world's richest nation is under-developed. Poverty, slums, health problems, lagging education pose major challenges for U.S. . . . the country is being told that 45 million Americans are poor, with 30 million of them described by the Government as poverty-stricken.

> *U.S. News & World Report*
> May 13, 1968

* On April 22, 1968, the prestigious Citizens Board of Inquiry into Hunger and Malnutrition in the United States made public a summary of the findings of an extensive study it had initiated a year before. "We have found concrete evidence," reported co-chairman Leslie Dunbar, "of chronic hunger and malnutrition in every part of the United States where we have held hearings or conducted field trips." Dunbar reported that at least 10,000,000 Americans were suffering from hunger and malnutrition.

The findings of the Citizens Board of Inquiry were published in a book entitled Hunger USA.

WASHINGTON, June 4 (AP)—The Commerce Department said today that the nation experienced a pronounced decline in poverty in the seven years that ended in 1966 . . .

> *New York Times*
> June 5, 1968

The House Agriculture Committee has not been able to find a single instance of starvation in the United States, it reported today.

There are many reports of malnutrition, it conceded, but these were attributed to local custom and ignorance.*

> Joseph A. Loftus
> *New York Times*
> June 17, 1968

Let me give you the promise of the future . . . Prosperity without war, progress without inflation.

> Richard M. Nixon, campaign speech
> Quoted in *Newsweek*
> November 4, 1968

No achievement gives me greater pride than the advances in the war on poverty.

> President Johnson
> Economic Report to Congress
> January 16, 1969

The infant mortality rate in the United States is higher than in 14 other countries . . . and in America's ghettoes and rural slums the death rate for black infants is actually increasing. An infant born to poor parents in the United States is twice as likely as his

---

* On December 22, 1970, Tom Wicker of the New York Times *quoted the Chairman of the House Agriculture Committee, Congressman W. R. Poage of Texas, as stating: "You know what happens in the beehive. They kill those drones. This is what happens in most primitive societies. Maybe we've just gotten too far away from the situation of primitive man."*

114

middle-class counterpart to die before reaching his first birthday.
. . . Many factors in the syndrome of poverty contribute to this
mortality rate . . . but experts point to malnutrition as a key
cause.

> Nick Kotz
> *Let Them Eat Promises—The Politics of Hunger
> in America,* 1970

How many is the time that my friends have pointed a finger
and said, "Look at that dumb Negro!" The charge is too often accurate. He is dumb, because we have denied him food. Dumb in
infancy, he has been blighted for life. . . .

I know that as a public official I am late to this problem. . . .
As a governor of South Carolina I had to put first things first.
There were many able-bodied standing around looking for jobs.
So, industrial development plus state pride resulted in the public
policy of covering up hunger. . . .

Let me categorically state there is hunger in South Carolina. I
have seen it with my own eyes. . . . Those weakened and diseased from hunger are dying from the disease caused by hunger.
Weakened and diseased, they become emotionally blind. . . .
The hunger and burden of the poor can no longer be ignored.

> Senator Ernest F. Hollings
> Hearing before
> Senate Select Committee on Nutrition
> February 19, 1969

PRESIDENT NIXON: The most troublesome question is, how wide
is the hunger problem in fact?

SECRETARY OF AGRICULTURE CLIFFORD HARDIN: We know there
are six million persons in families with less than $300 per capita
income, 25 million with less than $3,000 family income, and prob-
ably one half have nutritional problems, give or take one or two
million. We're absolutely convinced this is a serious problem . . .

PRESIDENT NIXON: To what extent does our report respond to the Senate [McGovern] hearings?* . . .

SECRETARY OF HEALTH, EDUCATION AND WELFARE ROBERT FINCH: Let's take the play away from the McGovern committee and send a couple of your guys [White House aides] in a helicopter to southern Virginia, for example.

PRESIDENT NIXON: Good. . . . How soon do we have to move? This week?

SECRETARY HARDIN: I have three speeches to give this week . . . And what I need to do when I speak is to say that I'm speaking within the policy of this Administration.

PRESIDENT NIXON: You can say that this Administration will have the first complete, far-reaching attack on the problem of hunger in history. Use all the rhetoric, so long as it doesn't cost money.

> From the official minutes of a White House meeting
> of members of the
> President's Urban Affairs Council
> Quoted in *Let Them Eat Promises*, by Nick Kotz
> March 17, 1969

The moment is at hand to put an end to hunger in America itself for all time.

> President Nixon
> Washington, D.C.
> May 6, 1969

Thirty million of our people live in poverty in the midst of plenty, even though our gross national product is approximately $1000 billion. Children are growing up in America with twisted minds and bodies because of malnutrition.

> Walter Reuther, Hearings
> before Joint Economic Subcommittee
> June 9, 1969

* *President Nixon was referring to the hearings being held before the Senate Select Committee on Nutrition and Human Needs under the chairmanship of Senator George McGovern.*

WASHINGTON—More than one-third of all Americans 65 years old and over live in poverty or near-poverty, a Senate committee was told today.

Senator Harrison Williams (D.–N.J.) said that for 7 million Americans who are both old and poor, food is treated as a luxury, an expendable which must give way in the face of other expenses.

San Francisco Examiner
September 9, 1969

We can control inflation without an increase in unemployment.
President Nixon
State of the Union Message
January 22, 1970

The economic situation is in control, our policies are working, and we are going to continue these policies.
Harold C. Passer
Assistant Secretary of Commerce for Economic Affairs
May 26, 1970

BIG BOARD SINKS TO A 7-YEAR LOW
DOW FALLS BY 20.81 IN LARGEST ONE-DAY DECLINE
SINCE THE DEATH OF PRESIDENT KENNEDY
New York Times
May 26, 1970

RATE OF JOBLESS UP TO 5% FOR MAY,
HIGHEST SINCE '65
New York Times
June 6, 1970

Our patience is being rewarded. The orthodox policies of this Administration are working.

> Secretary of the Treasury David M. Kennedy,
> addressing Joint Economic Committee
> July 21, 1970

. . . The Administration could use considerably better-looking data to go with its rhetoric. The cost of living in New York City rose at an annual rate of 7.2 percent in June, or 6 percent when seasonally adjusted. Nationally, the June rise in consumer prices was at an annual rate of 4.8 percent. . . .

. . . The Administration itself cautions that unemployment will probably continue to rise.

> Editorial
> *New York Times*
> June 22, 1970

QUESTION: Is the nation in a recession?

SECRETARY OF THE TREASURY KENNEDY: I don't know what "recession" means. If you define it for me, maybe I can answer your question. We are now in a period of adjustment.

> News Conference
> September 30, 1970
> San Francisco, California

RATE OF JOBLESS GOES UP TO 5.5%
New York Times
October 3, 1970

AMARILLO, Tex., Oct. 12—Vice President Agnew said tonight that a basic reason for unrest in the country was that Americans never had it so good.

118

"The hidden cause of malaise in America is the success—the success—of the American system," the Vice President emphasized. . . .

James M. Naughton
New York Times
October 13, 1970

4.6 MILLION UNEMPLOYED;
RATE HIGHEST IN 7½ YEARS
New York Times
December 5, 1970

I have become increasingly appalled to read of a country which during the past two decades has dropped from seventh in the world to sixteenth in the prevention of infant mortality; in female life expectancy from sixth to eighth; in male life expectancy from tenth to twenty-fourth. . . .

The country I am talking about is our own U.S.A., the home of the free, the home of the brave, and the home of a decrepit, inefficient, high-priced system of medical care.

. . . On the evidence we are clearly moving in the wrong direction; failing to secure for all our people the first right set down in the Declaration of Independence—the right to life.

From a speech by Thomas J. Watson, Jr.
Chairman of the Board
International Business Machines
Quoted in the *New York Times*
December 19, 1970

JOBLESS RATE RISES AGAIN;
MARCH LEVEL REACHES 6%
New York Times
April 3, 1971

119

13

O Master
Let Me Walk With Thee

*In which, amid claims of liberty and justice for all,
a dark skin is cause for oppression*

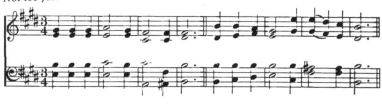

So I ask you tonight to join me and march along the road . . .
that leads to the Great Society, where no child will go unfed
. . . ; where every human being has dignity and every worker
has a job; where education is blind to color and employment is
unaware of race . . .

President Johnson
New York, N.Y.
May 28, 1964

Senate passage of the civil rights bill . . . goes further to invest the rights of man with the protection of the law than any legislation in this century.

President Johnson
Washington, D.C.
June 19, 1964

EXPERTS IDENTIFY MISSISSIPPI BODIES AS RIGHTS AIDES*

New York Times
August 6, 1964

. . . Some 40 churches have been burned or bombed in Mississippi in the past six months. . . .

Acts of violence have been erupting across the whole of Mississippi . . . In Vicksburg, a dynamite explosion damaged a church building early Sunday morning. In Meridian, a shotgun blast was fired into a Negro church where civil rights workers were sleeping Saturday night. In McComb, there have been 17 bombings, 9 beatings and four church burnings since June.

Editorial
New York Times
October 6, 1964

Civil rights cases handled by the FBI during fiscal year 1964 . . . received thorough, impartial attention . . .

FBI annual report
October, 1964

The FBI's 1964 annual report devotes one chapter to the domestic Communist menace but only one-third of a page to civil rights. . . . The report makes no mention of white terrorist organizations and indicates no FBI effort to infiltrate these as it does the Com-

---

* *The three civil rights workers who had been murdered were James Chaney, 21; Andrew Goodman, 20; and Michael Schwerner, 24.*

munist and liberal organizations. There is no reference to the
bombings that have destroyed dozens of Negro churches and
homes nor any indication of FBI activity under the federal anti-
bombing law.

> I.F. *Stone's Weekly*
> November 2, 1964

WASHINGTON—FBI Director J. Edgar Hoover yesterday called the
Rev. Martin Luther King, Jr., winner of the 1964 Nobel Peace
Prize, "the most notorious liar in the country."

> Times-Post Service
> *San Francisco Chronicle*
> November 19, 1964

If I hit him [Reverend Martin Luther King's aide] I don't know
it. One of the first things I ever learned was not to hit a nigger
with your fist because his head is too hard. Of course, the camera
might make me out a liar.

> Sheriff James G. Clark
> Selma, Alabama
> February 16, 1965

The call has gone out from the [civil rights] demonstration
leaders for every left-wing, pro-Communist fellow traveler and
Communist in the country to be here. . . .

> Governor George Wallace
> Montgomery, Alabama
> March 8, 1965

ALABAMA POLICE USE GAS AND CLUBS
TO ROUT NEGROES
57 ARE INJURED AT SELMA
AS TROOPS BREAK UP RIGHTS WALK IN MONTGOMERY

> *New York Times*
> March 8, 1965

CLERGYMAN DIES OF SELMA BEATING

SELMA, Ala., March 11—The Rev. James L. Reeb, the 38-year-old Boston minister who was beaten by whites here Tuesday night, died in the University of Alabama Hospital in Birmingham tonight.

> John Herbers
> *New York Times*
> March 12, 1965

. . . the cries of pain, and the hymns and protests of oppressed people, have summoned into convocation all the majesty of this great Government, this Government of the greatest nation on earth.

Our mission is at once the oldest and the most basic of this country: to right wrong, to do justice, to serve man.

> President Johnson
> addressing joint session of Congress
> March 15, 1965

WHITE RIGHTS WORKER IS SLAIN

MONTGOMERY, Ala., March 25— . . . A white woman worker for the Southern Christian Leadership conference was shot to death tonight while returning to Montgomery from Selma, Ala., where she had delivered a carload of civil rights workers who took part in the Freedom March that ended here today.

The victim was Mrs. Viola Gregg Liuzzo, 38 years old. . . .

> Paul L. Montgomery
> *New York Times*
> March 26, 1965

It is still safer on Highway 80 [the road on which Mrs. Liuzzo was shot] than it is riding a subway in New York.

> Governor Wallace
> NBC-TV "Today" Program
> March 26, 1965

WHITE SEMINARIAN SLAIN IN ALABAMA:
DEPUTY IS CHARGED

RIGHTS WORKER IS CUT DOWN BY SHOTGUN BLAST
AT STORE—PRIEST WITH HIM HURT—
VICTIMS SHOT WHILE WALKING WITH NEGRO GIRLS
AFTER ALL WERE FREED FROM JAIL

New York Times
August 21, 1965

Earlier in the spring, I asked the very able and dedicated Vice President, who has given his life to protecting equality among all races and religions and regions, to head up a blue-ribbon Cabinet task force to see what we could do about two million youngsters, most of whom came from broken homes . . . all of whom were without jobs, without education, without food. . . . We said we must get 500,000 jobs for these young people this summer. . . . The Vice President undertook this assignment. . . . He's placed 800,000 . . . and I am going to tell him, "Let's go to one million."

So the unemployment of young people has taken a nose dive. The employment has skyrocketed.

President Johnson
White House Conference on
Equal Employment Opportunity
August 20, 1965

Humphrey had reported at the conference's opening session Aug. 19 that non-whites had an unemployment rate twice that of whites. . . . "In fact, non-whites still experience the crisis condition of the Great Depression," Humphrey said. "Today, because of poor job opportunities, the median income of non-white families compared to whites is lower than it was a decade ago. It is only half as large. . . . In July . . . the nation's unemployment rate fell to 4.5%. . . . But for adult non-whites, the unemployment rate actually increased."

Facts on File
August 19-25, 1965

When you keep telling people they are unfairly treated and teach them disrespect for the law, you must expect this kind of thing sooner or later. . . .

One person threw a rock and, like monkeys in a zoo, others started throwing rocks.

> Police Chief William H. Parker
> commenting on the riots in
> Watts, Los Angeles, California
> August 12, 1965

If they're determined to set up anarchy, we're determined to confront them with sufficient force to prevent it.

> Mayor Sam Yorty
> Los Angeles, California
> August 14, 1965

For years a Los Angeles race explosion has been forecast . . . by sober civil rights workers all over the United States.

It was inevitable, they said, that pressures would build up here in this sprawling black ghetto. . . .

There is de facto segregation in schools, in libraries, in parks, in churches. Watts and its environs is a black world, with slums and indifferent education and limited opportunities.

> *San Francisco Chronicle*
> August 14, 1965

In the summer of 1964, Negro communities in seven eastern cities were stricken by riots. . . . The fundamental causes were largely the same:

Not enough jobs to go around . . .

Not enough schooling designed to meet the special needs of the disadvantaged Negro child, whose environment from infancy onward places him under a serious handicap.

A resentment, even hatred of the police, as a symbol of authority.

125

These riots were each a symptom of a sickness in the center of our cities.°

Violence in the City—A Report by the
Governor's Commission on the Los Angeles Riots
December 2, 1965

Some of these people that came in here [staff members of Dr. Martin Luther King's Southern Christian Leadership Conference] had no other purpose than to bring disorder to the streets. . . . They have been talking for the last year of violence . . . and instructing people in how to conduct violence. . . . They're responsible in large measure for the riots here.

Mayor Richard J. Daley
Chicago, Illinois
July 15, 1966

King had tried during the riot . . . to stem the disturbances. He had met July 14 with 100 clergymen and nuns; then the group had walked through the West Side, pleading for non-violence.

Facts on File
July 14-20, 1966

QUESTION: Mr. President, there seems to be an argument running over how much this country spends to rebuild the cities. What do you think the country can afford?

PRESIDENT JOHNSON: Well, we can afford whatever must be done. This Administration has done more than any Administration in the history of the country.

White House Press Conference
August 24, 1966

° "Rates of unemployment for non-white groups run twice as high as those for whites," reported the London Economist on July 15, 1967. "Even these figures underestimate the problem in the slum ghettos; last autumn a study by the Department of Labour found unemployment there three times as great as that in the country as a whole. A quarter to a third of the non-white teen-agers cannot find work. No wonder there are riots."

The Executive Reorganization Subcommittee of the Senate Operations Committee held hearings in Washington Aug. 15–Sept. 1 on the problems of the cities. . . .

Senator Robert F. Kennedy . . . testified Aug. 15 that the "most immediate and pressing" city problem was the plight of Negroes in the center of the city . . . "Unless the deprivation and alienation of the ghetto are eliminated," he said, "there is no hope for the city." . . .

Omaha Mayor A. V. Sorensen said one of the causes of rioting was that the promises of well-publicized federal programs had not been achieved. He testified that he had been unable after 15 months effort to get a single low-income housing unit built. . . .

[Senator] Ribicoff criticized the Administration's lack of planning and coordination for urban programs.

> *Facts on File*
> September 8–14, 1966

Vice President Humphrey last night called the summer's race riots the product of "a small but aroused minority . . . misled by demagogues into seeing its only outlet in anarchy and violence."

> Homer Bigart
> *New York Times*
> September 19, 1967

The drive for Negro revolution in this country is moving toward a climax. . . .

The forces which have shaped, molded and influenced this drive, and which now to a very substantial extent control it, have plans which involve major racial disturbances, of riot proportions, in some 20 cities of this country next year. . . .

The primary objective is acquisition of power by the Communists.

> Senator James O. Eastland
> Washington, D.C.
> October 12, 1967

The increasing prominence of the black power concept during 1967 "created a climate of unrest and has come to mean to many Negroes the 'power' to riot, burn, loot and kill," [J. Edgar Hoover] added.

New York Times
January 6, 1968

The summer of 1967 again brought racial disorders to American cities . . .

What happened? Why did it happen? . . .

This is our basic conclusion: Our nation is moving toward two societies, one black, one white—separate and unequal.

. . . Discrimination and segregation have long permeated much of American life . . .

Segregation and poverty have created in the racial ghetto a destructive environment totally unknown to most white Americans.

. . . White institutions created it, white institutions maintain it, and white society condones it. . . .

White racism is essentially responsible for the explosive mixture which has been accumulating in our cities since the end of World War II.*

Report of the National Advisory
Commission on Civil Disorders
February 29, 1968

MARTIN LUTHER KING IS SLAIN IN MEMPHIS**
New York Times
April 5, 1968

* The Report noted: "Between 2 and 2.5 million Negroes—16 to 20 percent of the total Negro population of all central cities—live in squalor and deprivation in ghetto neighborhoods.
** A biography of Georgia Governor Lester G. Maddox published in July 1968, The Riddle of Lester Maddox, by Bruce Galphin, related—according to the New York Times—that when tens of thousands of mourners marched in Dr. King's funeral in Atlanta the Governor told armed state troopers that if the marchers tried to enter Georgia's Capitol they should "shoot them down and stack them up."

The death rate of non-whites is 45 percent higher than that of whites of the same age—and life expectancy at birth is seven years shorter.

U.S. News & World Report
May 13, 1968

Black Americans . . . want the pride and self respect and the dignity which can come only if they have an equal chance to . . . have a piece of the action in the exciting ventures of private enterprise.

Former Vice President Nixon
Presidential Nomination Acceptance Speech
Miami Beach, Florida
August 8, 1968

When I finish this campaign, Negroes are going to know that my heart is in the right place and they are going to respect me.

Richard M. Nixon
Miami Beach, Florida
August 9, 1968

WASHINGTON, Oct. 13—Gov. Spiro T. Agnew asserted today that the nation could not allow protest demonstrations such as the Montgomery bus boycott because they let the individuals decide which laws they will obey or break.

New York Times
October 14, 1968

WASHINGTON, Oct. 15—The Southern Regional Council reported today there had been a "deplorable degree of failure" in desegregating Southern schools.

Pointing out that the public cry today is for "law and order," the council charged that "lawlessness and disorder" have been "rampant across the South" during 14 years of school desegregation efforts.

Marjorie Hunter
New York Times
October 16, 1968

To some extent, if you've seen one city slum you've seen them all.

Governor Agnew,
explaining why he had visited no Negro ghettos
during his campaign.
Detroit, Michigan
October 18, 1968

My task force on education pointed up that I was not considered . . . as a friend by many of our black citizens in America. . . . I can only say that by my actions as President I hope to rectify that. . . . I hope that I can gain the respect and I hope eventually the friendship of black citizens.

President Nixon
Washington, D.C.
February 6, 1969

BLACK RATIO ONLY 1 IN 50

A new study of black enrollments in 80 predominately white state universities shows that less than two of every 100 students, one of every 100 graduates and one of every 100 faculty members are American Negroes.

San Francisco Examiner & Chronicle
May 18, 1969

This Administration is unequivocally committed to the goal of finally ending racial discrimination in schools, steadily and speedily, in accordance with the law of the land.

From statement issued jointly by
Secretary of Health, Education and Welfare
Robert H. Finch and Attorney General
John N. Mitchell,
July 3, 1969

Civil rights lawyers in the Justice Department decided to protest the Nixon Administration desegregation policies after they were told by their superiors that political pressures had prompted the Government to call for a delay in the Mississippi school integration.

Fred P. Graham
New York Times
August 28, 1969

U.S. RIGHTS PANEL CRITICIZES NIXON ON DESEGREGATION—"MAJOR RETREAT" SEEN
New York Times
September 13, 1969

Extremist all-Negro, hate-type organizations, such as the Black Panther party, continue to fan the flames of riot and revolution in 1969.

J. Edgar Hoover
Summary of FBI Operations, 1969

The American Civil Liberties Union charged today that police across the country were conducting a campaign of "harrassment" against Black Panthers that seriously violated their civil rights.

The organization said that . . . high national officials including Vice President Spiro T. Agnew, Attorney General John N. Mitchell and FBI Director J. Edgar Hoover "by their statements and actions, have helped to create the climate of oppression and have encouraged local police to initiate the crackdown."

UPI Dispatch
December 29, 1969

In quantitative terms, which are reliable, the Negro is making extraordinary progress. . . .

131

The time may have come when the issue of race could benefit from a period of "benign neglect."

> Daniel Patrick Moynihan,
> counselor to President Nixon,
> in a memorandum to the President
> February 28, 1970

A Negro congressman said yesterday that President Nixon's "retreat" on civil rights has created an alienation "as deep as it is dangerous" between the President and America's Negroes. . . .

Representative William L. Clay (Dem–Mo.), saying he spoke for the other eight black House members, made the charge in complaining that Negro House members have been trying unsuccessfully for three months to see Mr. Nixon to try to heal this situation.

> *San Francisco Chronicle*
> May 19, 1970

CINCINNATI, June 29—The Nixon Administration was denounced as anti-Negro here tonight by the chairman of the board of the racially moderate National Association for the Advancement of Colored People.

"This is the first time since 1920," Bishop Stephen G. Spottswood said, "that the national Administration has made it a matter of calculated policy to work against the needs and aspirations of the largest minority of its citizens.

> Earl Caldwell
> *New York Times*
> June 30, 1970

Daniel Patrick Moynihan, counselor to President Nixon, has suggested that Negro-white relations are "getting better." . . .

His definition for "getting better" in race relations was "moving away from a past of racism and caste exclusion."

Peter Kihss
New York Times
July 4, 1970

WASHINGTON, Oct. 12—The United States Commission on Civil Rights said today that there had been a "major breakdown" in enforcement of the vast complex of Federal laws and executive orders against discrimination.

The finding . . . was based on a six-month study of the executive departments and agencies charged with enforcement of the body of civil rights law.

"The credibility of the Government's total civil rights effort has been seriously undermined," said [commission chairman] Father Hesburgh. . . .

John Herbers
New York Times
October 13, 1970

I happen to believe that there are no second-class citizens in America.

President Nixon
Tallahassee, Florida
October 28, 1970

14

O Sons and Daughters

*In which, for protesting the sins of their fathers,
the sons are accused of being sinners*

With feeling

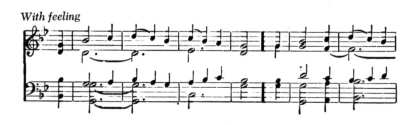

One of the most alarming aspects of these student demonstrations is the ever-present evidence that the guiding hand of Communists and extreme leftists was involved.

> *The Police Chief,*
> official publication of
> International Association of Chiefs of Police
> April 1965

You've got a few hundred—a thousand at most . . . who have triggered, organized and led the so-called "demonstrations" [at the University of California, Berkeley].

. . . In my opinion they are not legitimate, genuine students at all. Many of them are what you might call fugitives, from Eastern and Midwestern colleges and universities, who have been in trouble before. Now they are at Berkeley to cause trouble. . . .

Dr. Max Rafferty,
California State Superintendent of Public Instruction,
interview in *U.S. News & World Report*
May 17, 1965

The students, intellectuals, university professors and others who stage "teach-ins" and demonstrate from New York to San Francisco . . . have a right to be heard in a land with our traditions. We are engaged in an unpopular and unnecessary war.

John S. Knight, publisher of the Knight newspapers
Detroit Free Press,
October 24, 1965

DANANG, South Vietnam—FBI Director J. Edgar Hoover has assured a fighting young Marine lieutenant here that anti-Vietnam demonstrators in the U.S. represent a minority "for the most part composed of halfway citizens who are neither morally, mentally nor emotionally mature. This is true whether the demonstrator be the college professor or the beatnik."

Scripps-Howard newspapers,
November 1, 1965

Put away all the childish divisive things, if you want the maturity and the unity that is the mortar of a nation's greatness.

I do not think that those men who are out there fighting for us tonight think we should enjoy the luxury of fighting each other back home.

President Johnson
Chicago, Illinois
May 17, 1966

I am to report to Oakland, California, September 13, to leave for Vietnam. My position on my orders is simply no. I will not be used any longer. My fighting is back home in Philadelphia's ghettos where I was born and raised. I will not be sent 10,000 miles away from home to be used as a tool of the aggressors of the Vietnamese people. . . . I think most of the guys in my company support what I am doing. But they are afraid to take a stand, so I am asking for the support of all people all over the nation and especially black people . . . to join me and support me in my struggle.

> Private Ronald Lockman,
> addressing the New Politics Convention,
> Chicago, Illinois
> August 31, 1967

Here we are, the way politics ought to be in America. The politics of happiness . . . the politics of joy . . . and that's the way it's going to be from here on out.

> Vice President Humphrey
> Washington, D.C.
> April 27, 1968

CHICAGO, August 29— . . . Mayor Richard J. Daley defended today the manner in which anti-war, anti-Humphrey demonstrations were suppressed in downtown Chicago last night.

Mr. Daley described the demonstrators as "terrorists" and said they had come here determined to "assault, harrass and taunt the police into reacting before television cameras." . . .

In an interview tonight on the Columbia Broadcasting System television network, the Mayor said he had "intelligence reports" indicating that persons who he did not identify had planned to assassinate him, the three leading Presidential candidates and others. He gave no further details.

> R.W. Apple, Jr.
> *New York Times*
> August 30, 1968

People were led to believe that the police waded in without provocation. . . . We ought to quit pretending that Mayor Daley did something that was wrong. He didn't condone a thing that was wrong. He tried to protect lives.

Vice President Humphrey
Minneapolis, Minnesota
August 31, 1968

During the week of the Democratic National Convention, the Chicago police were the targets of mounting provocation both by word and act. . . .

. . . The nature of the response was unrestrained and indiscriminate police violence on many occasions, particularly at night.

That violence . . . was often inflicted upon persons who had broken no law, disobeyed no order, made no threat. These included peaceful demonstrators, onlookers, and large numbers of residents who were simply passing through, or happened to live in the areas where confrontations were occurring.

Newsmen and photographers were singled out for assault and their equipment deliberately damaged. . . .

Chicago Study Team report,
Rights in Conflict,
November 18, 1968[*]

NEW YORK, Sept. 6— . . . The Republican Vice Presidential candidate [Spiro Agnew] told a news conference here that he saw a "definite link" between the campus revolt and Communists.

. . . He said that after watching the evolution of student disorders in the United States . . . he had reached the conclusion

---

[*] *Among the data cited by the Study Team as indicative of the attitude of the police was an excerpt from the tape of the Chicago Police Department radio log:—*

Police Car Operator: "Get a wagon over at 1436. We've got an injured hippie."

These remarks from four other police cars follow: "That's no emergency." "Let him take a bus." "Kick the fucker." "Knock his teeth out."

137

that they revolved basically around the "sort of person willing to be identified with Communist causes."

Homer Bigart
New York Times
September 7, 1968

In all, about a hundred students were hurt at Columbia University. . . . The police simply ran wild. Those who tried to say they were innocent bystanders or faculty were given the same flailing treatment as the students. For most of the students it was their first encounter with brutality and blood, and they responded in fear and anger. The next day, almost the entire campus responded to a call for a student strike. In a few hours, thanks to the New York City Police Department, a large part of the Columbia campus had become radicalized.

Daniel Bell,
"Columbia and the New Left"
The Public Interest
Fall 1968

SANTA BARBARA, Calif., Sept. 15—Richard M. Nixon contended today that he was becoming a favorite of America's young people . . .

New York Times
September 16, 1968

What I'm saying to you is we're just kind of sick and tired of having this country run down by a group of phony intellectuals who don't understand what we mean by hard work and patriotism.

Spiro Agnew
Woodbridge, New Jersey
October 14, 1968

The present generation of young people in our universities is the best informed, the most intelligent and the most idealistic this country has ever known. . . .

The ability, social consciousness and conscience, political sensitivity, and honest realism of today's students take seriously ideals taught in schools and churches, and often at home, and then they see a system that denies its ideals in actual life. Racial injustice and the war in Vietnam stand out as prime illustrations of our society's deviation from its professed ideals and the slowness with which the system reforms itself.

> *Crisis at Columbia:*
> *Report of the Fact-Finding*
> *Commission Appointed to*
> *Investigate the Disturbance at Columbia University*
> *in April and May 1968*
> Vintage Books, 1968

I believe in youthful dissent. I believe in young people wanting change.

> Governor Ronald Reagan
> Sacramento, California
> January 5, 1969

I am determined that academic freedom and the pursuit of knowledge will be upheld, protected and preserved.

> Governor Ronald Reagan
> Sacramento, California
> January 7, 1969

SHOTGUNS AND TEAR GAS DISPERSE RIOTERS
NEAR THE BERKELEY CAMPUS
> *New York Times*
> May 16, 1969

Last Tuesday I was gassed twice in Berkeley. . . . The police and National Guard . . . are using a chemical called CS . . . that the Army uses in Vietnam. . . .

Many other people, of course, got hurt far worse than I did. They were clubbed and shot as well as gassed. One 25-year-old onlooker was killed by a buckshot pellet the size of a marble. . . .

In Berkeley, under cover of Governor Reagan's three-month-old "state of emergency," police have . . . gone on a riot displaying a lawless brutality . . . along with . . . the firing of buckshot at fleeing crowds and unarmed bystanders, and the gassing—at times for no reason at all—of entire streets and portions of a college campus.*

> Peter Barnes
> *Newsweek*
> June 2, 1969

In the past generation, since 1941, this nation has paid for fourteen years of peace with fourteen years of war. . . . Perhaps this is why my generation is so fiercely determined to pass on a different legacy. . . . We want to be remembered not as the generation that suffered in war, but as the generation that was tempered in the fire for a great purpose: to make the kind of peace that the next generation will be able to keep.

> President Nixon
> Colorado Springs, Colorado
> June 4, 1969

These students were educated to value truth and justice. . . . Now they see their own country is practicing injustice. Now their own country, try as it will, cannot force them to cooperate. . . .

---

* *In February 1970, twelve sheriff's deputies were indicted by a Federal Grand Jury for their actions during the May 1969 disturbances at Berkeley. Among the charges brought against the deputies were those of shooting persons with shotguns and beating others after their arrest. All the deputies were later exonerated.*

Johnson promised peace and we got war. Nixon promised peace and the generals say, "at least two more years of war." When will we have peace? When we are all dead?

> From a college student's letter
> quoted by Senator Fulbright,
> Hearing of the Joint Economic Committee,
> June 4, 1969

Young and old, we are all Americans, and if we are to remain free we must talk to each other, listen to each other, young and old alike. . . . NOW, THEREFORE, I, RICHARD NIXON, President of the United States of America, do hereby designate the period from September 28 to October 4, 1969, as National Adult-Young Communication Week.

> Proclamation signed by President Nixon
> at the White House
> September 25, 1969

. . . I understand that there has been and continues to be opposition to the war in Vietnam on the campuses and in the nation. As far as this activity is concerned, we expect it. However, under no circumstances will I be affected whatever by it.

> President Nixon
> Washington, D.C.
> September 26, 1969

. . . Mr. J. Edgar Hoover, in testimony before this commission [Cox Fact-Finding Commission Appointed to Investigate Disturbances at Columbia] on September 18, 1968 stated:

'Communists are in the forefront of civil rights, anti-war and student demonstrations, many of which ultimately become disorderly and erupt into violence. . . ."

> *The Politics of Protest*:
> *A Task Force Report Submitted to the*
> *National Commission on the Causes and Prevention*
> *of Violence,* by Jerome H. Skolnick, 1969

By contrast, a "blue-ribbon" investigating committee appointed by the Regents of the University of California concluded:

"We found no evidence that the FSM [Free Speech Movement at Berkeley] was organized by the Communist Party, the Progressive Labor movement, or any other outside group. . . ."

And more recently, the prestigious Cox Commission, which was headed by the former Solicitor General of the United States and investigated last spring's Columbia disturbances, reported:

"We reject the view that ascribes the April and May disturbances primarily to a conspiracy of student revolutionaries. . . ."

> Jerome H. Skolnick
> *The Politics of Protest,* 1969

Vice President Agnew tonight denounced last week's Vietnam Moratorium Day as an unwise demonstration "encouraged by an effete corps of impudent snobs who characterize themselves as intellectuals."

> Marjorie Hunter
> *New York Times*
> October 20, 1969

Vice President Agnew demonstrated a truly monumental insensitivity to the most profound concern of millions of Americans —and particularly the nation's youth—when he described last week's Vietnam Moratorium as the creation of "an effete corps of impudent snobs." . . . Idealistic young men and women from the nation's campuses were joined by Americans of every generation and from all walks of life in an urgent appeal that the United States Government follow a more effective path to peace.

. . . it is clear to all perceptive observers that American youth today is far more imbued with idealism, a sense of service and a deep humanitarianism than any generation in recent history, including Mr. Agnew's.

> Editorial
> *New York Times*
> October 21, 1969

WASHINGTON—FBI Director J. Edgar Hoover suggested yesterday that New Left and black militant groups are "encouraged and inflamed from without" in a violent campaign against the Government." . . . He sought to link the huge anti-war rally here last November 15 with "international Communist elements."

San Francisco Chronicle
January 3, 1970

ISLA VISTA, Calif., April 21—Kevin Moran was buried today as this college community started to unwind from five days of tension . . .

Mr. Moran was a 21-year-old senior here at the University of California's Santa Barbara campus. He was killed by a single bullet early Saturday morning while helping other students put out fires set by a band of marauding demonstrators.

After maintaining for several days that Mr. Moran had been shot by a sniper, Sheriff James Webster of Santa Barbara County announced yesterday that a policeman had accidentally fired his gun at the time the youth was struck.

Steven V. Roberts
New York Times
April 22, 1970

. . . In his speech at a Republican fund-raising dinner in Hollywood, Fla. [on April 28], the Vice President attacked acts of student violence at various universities and cited among them students at Cornell "who, wielding pipes and tire chains, beat a dormitory president into unconsciousness."

New York Times
April 30, 1970

No such incident has ever occurred at Cornell University. It is incredible that the Vice President of the United States should make such a public statement for which there is no basis in fact.

143

The damage you do through such irresponsible and widely publicized statements is irreparable.

From a telegram to Vice President Agnew
from Dale R. Corson,
President of Cornell University
April 29, 1970

You see these bums, you know, blowing up the campuses.
Listen, the boys on the college campuses today are the luckiest
people in the world—going to the greatest universities—and there
they are burning up the books. I mean storming around about
this issue. You name it. Get rid of the war, there'll be another one.

President Nixon, addressing Pentagon employees
Washington, D.C.
May 1, 1970

I think we are up against the strongest, well-trained militant
revolutionary group that has ever been assembled in America.
. . . We are going to use every weapon possible.

Governor James Rhodes
Kent, Ohio
May 3, 1970

4 KENT STATE STUDENTS KILLED BY TROOPS
KENT, Ohio, May 4—Four students at Kent State University, two
of them women, were shot to death this afternoon by a volley of
National Guard gunfire. At least 8 other students were wounded.

John Kifner
New York Times
May 5, 1970

In Columbus, Sylvester Del Corso, Adjutant General of the
Ohio National Guard, said in a statement that the guardsmen had
been forced to fire after a sniper opened fire against the troops
from 'a nearby rooftop . . .

Frederick P. Wenger, the Assistant Adjutant General, said the troops had opened fire after they were shot at by a sniper.

John Kifner
New York Times
May 5, 1970

KENT, Ohio, May 5—Officials of the Ohio National Guard said today they were unable to produce evidence of sniper fire at the guardsmen who killed the four Kent State students here yesterday.

John Kifner
New York Times
May 6, 1970

She resented being called a "bum" because she disagreed with someone else's opinion. She felt the war in Cambodia was wrong. Is this dissent a crime? Is this a reason for killing her? Have we come to such a state in this country that a young girl has to be shot because she disagrees deeply with the actions of her government?

Arthur Krause,
father of Allison Krause,
student killed at Kent State University,
Quoted in *New York Times*
May 7, 1970

WASHINGTON, May 6—In an extraordinary letter of protest, Secretary of the Interior Walter J. Hickel complained to President Nixon today that the Administration was turning its back on the great mass of American youth and thereby contributing to anarchy and revolt.

145

Mr. Hickel warned that further attacks by Vice President Agnew on the motives of young Americans would solidify their hostility beyond the reach of reason. . . .

> Max Frankel
> *New York Times*
> May 7, 1968

Cool it, Wally, this will blow over in twenty-four hours.

> A Nixon aide, as quoted by
> Secretary of the Interior, Walter Hickel,
> Associated Press, May 13, 1970

Is this just a ferment of youth? Are these young people just showing their idealism? Or is it possible that there is a plot involved? Is it possible that some people set out several years ago to make this happen?

> Governor Ronald Reagan
> Sacramento, California
> May 12, 1970

JACKSON, Miss., May 15—A barrage of police gunfire that lasted 30 seconds and consisted of 140 shots left two students dead and nine other persons wounded here last night. All the dead and wounded were Negroes.

> Roy Reed
> *New York Times*
> May 16, 1970

JACKSON, Miss., June 5 (AP)—Gov. John Bell Williams says that a state investigation showed the police acted in self-defense in killing two young Negroes in a confrontation with students May 15 at Jackson State College.

In a television report last night, the Governor said that policemen were fired on by snipers before firing . . .

> *New York Times*
> June 6, 1970

WASHINGTON, June 9 (AP)—The man heading the Government's investigation of student deaths on the Kent State and Jackson State campuses says there is "insufficient evidence" to support officials' allegations of sniper fire.

"We have at this time insufficient evidence to establish the presence of a sniper," Assistant Attorney General Jerris Leonard said of the May 15 deaths of two black youths in a fusillade of police bullets at Jackson State College in Mississippi.*

> *New York Times*
> June 10, 1970

NIXON IS ADVISED TO HEED STUDENTS
DR. HEARD, HEAD OF PANEL ON CAMPUS UNREST,
PRAISES THE MOTIVES OF YOUTHS
New York Times
July 24, 1970

I'll tell you who's not informed . . . It's these stupid kids. Why, they don't know the issues. . . .

And the professors, they are just as bad if not worse. They don't know anything. Nor do these stupid bastards who are ruining our educational institutions.

> Attorney General Mitchell
> Washington, D.C.
> September 16, 1970

* In a statement on August 4, 1970, the national president of the Fraternal Order of Police, Sergeant John Harrington of the Philadelphia, Pa., Police Department, indicated what he felt was the prevailing attitude among policemen in many parts of the country. "Unless the courts stop their permissiveness," he said, "unless the people we work for are going to back us up, then the feeling of policemen is—maybe we better resort to the old Mexican deguello—a shootout in which we take no prisoners."

In the Holt, Rinehart and Winston Spanish-English dictionary deguello is defined as "throat cutting, massacre or slaughter."

Sergeant Harrington added that he viewed pop festivals as a "Communist plot to destroy our youth."

I am very proud to be called a pig. It stands for pride, integrity and guts.

Governor Reagan
Oroville, California
October 3, 1970

They should have shot all the troublemakers.

Seabury Ford, special prosecutor
Ohio Grand Jury investigating Kent State shootings
Quoted in interview in Akron *Beacon-Journal*,
October 24, 1970*

Seabury Ford was one of three special prosecutors appointed by Governor Rhodes to handle the Grand Jury, which brought in a report absolving the National Guard and Ohio authorities of any guilt in the killing of the four students and the wounding of nine others. The Grand Jury indicted 25 persons, mostly students and professors, linked with the anti-war demonstration.

The Scranton Commission and Justice Department investigations brought in different findings. According to these, the National Guard fired without any justification; there was no sniper fire whatsoever; and not one of the students killed or wounded had participated in any disorder in Kent.

15

Hark, the Herald Angels Sing

A chorale based on the gospel according to
Assistant Secretary of Defense Arthur Sylvester:
"Look, if you think any American official is
going to tell you the truth, then you're stupid." *

In unison; quietly and reverently

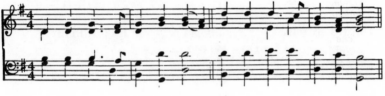

No facts have been withheld, and none are.
> Vice President Humphrey
> Hartford, Connecticut
> March 6, 1965

I don't know any subject on which the American public has been more informed than Vietnam.
> Secretary of State Rusk
> June 11, 1966

* *The conversation during which Assistant Secretary of Defense Sylvester made this remark took place with a group of American foreign correspondents in Saigon on July 17, 1965, and was reported by CBS correspondent Morely Safer in* Dateline 1966, *the publication of the Overseas Press Club of America.*

The freedom to know the truth—and let the truth make us free —must never be compromised or destroyed.

President Johnson
Chicago, Illinois
April 1, 1968

Let us begin by committing ourselves to the truth, to see it like it is and to tell it like it is, to find the truth, to speak the truth and live with the truth. That's what we will do.

Richard Nixon
Nomination acceptance speech
Miami, Florida
August 8, 1968

After all, what does a politician have but his credibility?

Governor Agnew
New York, N.Y.
August 23, 1968

I promise the truth shall be the policy of the Nixon-Agnew Administration.

Governor Agnew
San Francisco, California
September 20, 1968

I have tried to present the facts about Vietnam with complete honesty. And I shall continue to do so in my reports to the American people.

President Nixon
Washington, D.C.
May 15, 1969

I want to make sure that we open up no credibility gap.

Secretary of Defense Laird
Washington, D.C.
February 3, 1971

But can you believe this? I understand why this question is raised by many honest, sincere people.

President Nixon
Washington, D.C.
April 7, 1971

Amen

Epilogue

The inglorious record revealed in this book remains unconcluded.

Even as these lines are written, evidence of the continuing discrepancy between the words and the deeds of the nation's leaders mounts on every side. The term "Credibility Gap" inadequately defines this state of affairs. The essential question is not simply misrepresentation of the facts; it is, rather, misrepresentation of the people. The issues transcend those of truth and falsehood. At stake is our future. The Credibility Gap is a symptom of a malaise that imperils the life of the nation.

The devious domestic and foreign policies pursued by government leaders in recent years, and the camouflaging of the crucial actions to which they have committed the nation, have caused incalculable losses to the American people and the peoples of other lands. There are no scales in which to measure the bloodshed, misery and waste of man's wealth that have prevailed since the military-industrial complex came to shape the politics of our land.

When the *New York Times* brought to light the secret Pentagon Papers, some political leaders declared that their publication came close to treason. The highest form of treason, however, is not treason against governments but against the people who elect those governments. And one may ask: Which comes closer to treason—the publication of the Pentagon Papers, or the stratagems they disclose of top government officials and military leaders in involving this nation in an undeclared and calamitous war?

Which constitutes the greater betrayal—the betrayal of alleged military secrets by the press, or the betrayal of vital interests of the American people by their elected representatives?

Other questions too must now be asked: Why did falsities and delusions so multiply in this country during the Cold War years? To what extent are they responsible not only for catastrophe abroad but for the mounting social problems, and—with funds desperately needed to meet those problems—for the diversion of vast government expenditures into the coffers of the military-industrial complex?

Since the *Times* exposé, the air has become clamorous with the alibis of political figures who helped create the Credibility Gap and with their charges and countercharges. This cacophony will doubtless increase as the Presidential election draws near.

In considering the qualifications of candidates for government office in the approaching elections, American citizens might keep in mind these words of Thomas Paine: "When a man has so corrupted and prostituted the chastity of his mind as to subscribe his professional belief to things he does not believe, he has prepared himself for the commission of every other crime."

When a government ceases to reflect the interests of the people, and when in fact its members deliberately misguide the people on issues of crucial import, the time has come to change the composition of that government by electing to office true representatives of the people.

It is hoped that the record provided by this *Hymnal* will prove useful to concerned American citizens at this time.

A.E.K.

Note on Sources

The purpose of this note is not merely to supplement the documentation of the materials in the book but also, and especially, to provide the interested reader with sources which will enable him to conduct his own investigation into the workings of the Credibility Gap.

As indicated in the foreword, the *Hymnal* makes no claim to provide an exhaustive survey of the official falsities and delusions that have proliferated during the period of the Credibility Gap but rather offers a representative summary of them. A sizable encyclopedia would be needed to encompass them all.

The sources of the *Hymnal's* statements, headlines, and selections from newspaper articles and books are cited in the text, with the exception of certain direct quotations from public utterances of Government and other public officials. In the compilation of this material we also consulted various supplementary sources, both for the purpose of accumulating additional statements by public officials and of further establishing the falsity or veracity of the quotations in this book.

In the preparation of the book we made extensive reference to the Index of *The New York Times, Readers' Guide to Periodical Literature, Facts on File* and *Vital Speeches*. We also drew heavily on the Hearings and Reports of various U.S. Congressional Committees and the Reports of a number of official and public investigatory commissions.

Investigations by reporters for major newspapers and the television networks into various aspects of the Credibility Gap were an indispensable reference source; and we must acknowledge a special indebtedness to these reporters, many of whose names appear in this book. Of signal value also has been the reportage of such public television programs as "Newsroom," KQED, San Francisco.

Much material, as indicated in the text, has been taken from newspapers, magazines and other journals. One publication which contains vital material often not available in the general press, and to which we wish to record our appreciation in particular, is *I. F. Stone's Bi-Weekly* (4420 29th Street NW, Washington, D.C.).

The following summary of source references is by no means an exhaustive bibliography, being intended primarily as a record and acknowledgment of those sources we have found most useful, and as a guide to the interested reader.

A pioneer work dealing with Governmental deceits in domestic and foreign affairs during the initial stages of the Credibility Gap is *Anything But the Truth* by the Washington correspondents Erwin Knoll and William McGaffin (New York: Putnam, 1968). This work, the opening chapter of which was published in part in the September 1967 issue of *The Progressive* magazine under the title "The White House Lies," was the first book devoted to the subject of the Credibility Gap. An interesting compilation of evidence of Governmental deceits, covering the first years of the Johnson Administration and background material, appears in "Credibility Gaps and the Presidency" in the February 1968 issue of *Editorial Research Reports*.

There is of course a copious literature dealing with the war in Indochina which contains detailed evidence of official deceits and delusions. Among the books we found of special value in this regard are: *The United States in Vietnam* by George McTurnan Kahin and John W. Lewis (New York: Dial Press, 1967, revised edition, Dell Publishing Co., 1969); *In the Name of America,* Research Director, Seymour Melman (New York: Clergy and Laymen Concerned About Vietnam, 1968); *My Lai Four* by Seymour M. Hersh (New York: Random House, 1970); *Air War—Vietnam* by Frank Harvey (New York: Bantam Books, 1967); *America's Vietnam Policy—The Strategy of Deception* by Edward S. Herman and Richard B. Du Boff (Washington, D.C.: Public Affairs Press, 1966); *The Vietnam Reader,* edited by Marcus G. Raskin and Bernard B. Fall (New York: Vintage Books, 1965); *Vietnam North* by Wilfred Burchett (New York: International Publishers, 1966); *Vietnam! Vietnam!* by Felix Greene (Palo Alto, Cal.: Fulton Publishing Company, 1966); and *Vietnam and International Law,* issued by Lawyers Committee on American Policy Toward Vietnam (Flanders, N.J.: O'Hare Books, 1967). A revealing compilation of official statements, including many false and contradictory ones, is presented in *Quotations Vietnam: 1945-1970,* edited by William G. Effros (New York: Random House, 1970). Extensive evidence of misrepresentation of facts about the war by Government officials appears in the Hearings of the U.S. Senate Foreign Affairs Committee and the Hearings of the U.S. Senate Subcommittee on Refugees dealing with refugee and civilian war casualty problems in Indochina. (Reports of these Congressional hearings, and of others mentioned below, are available from the Government Printing Office, Washington, D.C.)

Of historic importance in evaluating the origins and nature of the war in Indochina—and the governmental deceptions and duplicities in its conduct—are the secret Pentagon Papers, which the *New York Times* began publishing on June 13, 1971.

For basic material on the military-industrial complex, and evidence of Governmental deceits and delusions during recent years in this area, these are among the more illuminating books: *Militarism, U.S.A.,* by Colonel James A. Donovan (New York: Charles Scribner's Sons, 1970); *Pentagon Capitalism—The Political Economy of War* by Seymour Melman (New York: McGraw-Hill Co., 1970); *The Weapons Culture* by Ralph Lapp (New York: W. W. Norton & Co., 1968); *The Economy of Death* by Richard J. Barnet (New York: Atheneum, 1969); *What Price Vigilance? The Burdens of National Defense* by Bruce M. Russett (New Haven and London: Yale University Press, 1970); and *The Ultimate Folly* by Richard D. McCarthy (New York: Alfred A. Knopf, 1969). An illuminating insight into the delusions of military leaders can be derived from *Design for Survival* by General Thomas S. Power (New York: Coward-McCann, 1965); *Neither Liberty nor Safety* by General Nathan Twining (New York: Holt, 1966); and *America Is in Danger* by General Curtis LeMay (New York: Funk & Wagnalls, 1968). The Hearings before the Senate Subcommittee on Economy in Government—especially those concerning the Military Budget and National Economic Priorities, the Economics of Military Procurement, and the Acquisition of Weapons Systems—are a vital source of material not only on the general workings of the military-industrial complex but also on what the Subcommittee Chairman, Senator William Proxmire, characterizes as the complex's "lies" and "deceptions."

Among the books containing significant evidence of Governmental deceits and delusions in recent years concerning the national economy and social problems in the United States are: *Let Them Eat Promises—The Politics of Hunger in America* by Nick Kotz (Englewood Cliffs, N.J.: Prentice-Hall, Inc., 1970); *The Shame of a Nation* by Philip Stern and George de Vincent (New York: Ivan Obolensky, Inc., 1965); *The Other America* by Michael Harrington (New York: The Macmillan Co., 1963); *In the Midst of Plenty* by Ben H. Bagdikian (Boston: Beacon Press, 1964); *Civil Rights and the American Negro,* edited by Albert P. Blaustein and Robert L. Zangrando (New York: Washington Square Press, 1968); *Race Relations in the USA, 1954-1968,* a Kessing's Research Report (New York: Charles Scribner's Sons, 1970); *The Negro in the 20th Century,* edited by John Hope Franklin and Isidore Starr (New York: Random House, 1967); and *Rivers of Blood, Years of Darkness* by Robert Conot (New York: Bantam Books, 1967). Valuable material can also be found in the Reports submitted to the National Commission on the Causes and Prevention of Violence—*Rights in Conflict,* prepared by Daniel Walker (New York: Bantam Books, 1968); *Violence in America,* prepared by Hugh Davis Graham and Ted Robert Gurr (New York: The New American Library, 1969); and *The Politics of Protest,* prepared by Jerome H. Skolnick (New York: Simon and Schuster, 1969). Also illuminating is the *Report of the National Advisory Commission on Civil Disorders* (New York: Bantam Books, 1968).

A.E.K.
S.J.K.
B.J.K.

About the Author

———————

ALBERT E. KAHN has earned an international reputation for his books exposing political intrigue and the machinations of men in high places. His book *Sabotage!*, dealing with Fascist conspiratorial activities, was one of the top best sellers of the Second World War; and his subsequent works on secret diplomacy and the Cold War era have been translated into more than twenty languages. During the McCarthy period, Mr. Kahn secured and published the sensational confession of the former McCarthy aide, Harvey Matusow, whose admissions of perjury as a paid government witness did much to destroy the professional-witness racket.

A writer of singular versatility, Mr. Kahn is also the author of *Days With Ulanova,* which was hailed as a work of major importance on the ballet. His most recent work was *Joys and Sorrows—Reflections by Pablo Casals, as told to Albert E. Kahn.* Permanent collections of his photographic studies of Ulanova and Casals are housed at the Museum and Library of the Performing Arts at Lincoln Center, New York, and at the San Francisco Museum of Art, respectively.

Born in London, England, Mr. Kahn is a graduate of Dartmouth College. He is married, has three sons, and lives in Glen Ellen, California.

Assisting Mr. Kahn in the research on *The Unholy Hymnal* were his sons—Steven Kahn, a graduate of San Francisco State College and a short-story writer, and Brian Kahn, a graduate of the University of California, Berkeley, who is currently attending Boalt Law School.